MINERALS

The Forgotten Nutrient

Your *Secret Weapon* for Getting and Staying Healthy

———

Joy Stephenson-Laws, JD

with Monya De, MD, MPH
Franz Gliederer, MD, MPH
Pauline J. Jose, MD

pH
Proactive Health™
Labs

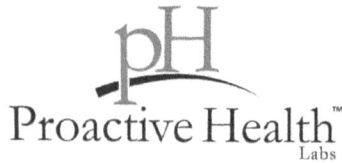

ABOUT PROACTIVE HEALTH LABS

Proactive Health Labs (pH) is a 501(c)(3) nonprofit health assessment and wellness organization committed to making sure you have the information and tools you need to get and stay your healthiest.

pH's philosophy is that the better educated you are about how to protect your health, the more benefits of a healthy life you will enjoy. And being more educated also allows you to better partner with your health care providers in making well-informed choices.

As part of pH's commitment to making sure you have all the education you need to proactively manage your health, you can find a substantial database of credible, research-based educational blogs at phlabs.org/healthinfo.

And for those who are facing challenging health issues – such as a new diagnosis, conflicting medical opinions or poor outcomes from treatment – pH offers patient advocacy for one-on-one support nationwide at phlabs.org/phpatientadvocates.

WHAT PEOPLE ARE SAYING

"Enjoyed the book very much and learned a ton. I think you have pointed out the importance of minerals, but also pointed out that too much of these individual minerals can have significant adverse effects. You also were appropriately cautious in raising the issues of altered metabolism seen in renal failure. I think the book will be popular, particularly for people who are very interested in living a healthy lifestyle. I think a minority of physicians who do not have a specific interest in nutrition are not aware of a considerable amount of the material that you presented. But, it will stimulate some conversation and education."

-Robert Kerlan, medical doctor

"This book does a great job of explaining the intricate relationships between the minerals in the body and the importance of maintaining optimal ratios in a way that is accessible to Joe Public, but that also addresses professionals. I just wish texts like this were required reading for medical, nutritional or any and all health care-related students and providers!"

-Melissa Ashworth Michelini, yoga instructor

"Very pertinent and an easy read to stress the importance of knowing our internal environment and being proactive in managing it for better health. This is the most comprehensive book I have ever read on minerals and their application to disease processes and health."

-Susan Acquisto, health care consultant

Printed in the United States of America
First Edition 2017

ISBN: 978-0-9978291-2-9

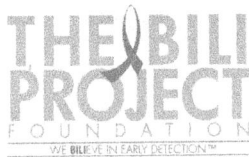

ABOUT THE BILI PROJECT FOUNDATION

The Bili Project Foundation's mission is to reduce the incidence and improve the outcome of hepatobiliary cancers, which are cancers of the liver, gallbladder or bile ducts (cholangiocarcinoma). The Bili Project promotes research to identify early signs and symptoms, as well as treatment options for this silent, fast-acting group of cancers.

The Bili Project Foundation was founded by Sue Acquisto, the wife of Vince Acquisto, and his business partner Joy Stephenson-Laws after Vince was diagnosed with and later passed from bile duct cancer. Bile duct cancer and other biliary system cancers are among the most difficult to detect. If screening or testing for risk factors or silent symptoms of this type of cancer had been available for Vince, perhaps he would have had a chance for successful treatment at an early stage. Inspired by Vince's passion for education, Sue and Joy partnered with the University of California San Francisco (UCSF) medical research team and other institutions to assess how to better stop this quick and silent killer.

As a result of this partnership began California's first Hepatobiliary Tissue Tumor Bank where UCSF and other collaborating institutions now have access to banked tumor samples in order to advance the research of these diseases. UCSF's Hepatobiliary Tissue Tumor Bank is now thriving and houses over a hundred tumor samples, all of which have the potential to lead to groundbreaking research in early detection, treatments and cures of these diseases.

DEDICATION

I dedicate this book to my mother, Gladys Young, and brother, Herman Ricketts, MD, who both taught me the importance of empowering myself through education.

- Joy Stephenson-Laws

CONTENTS

PART II
Minerals as Part of Your Proactive Health Plan

PART III
Your Lifestyle and Minerals

PART IV
pH Labs Editorial Board

PREFACE

The idea for this book about minerals came about while I was working with an incredible team of physicians. In discussing the importance of various nutrients such as carbohydrates, fats and protein, it became apparent that we knew relatively little about minerals. Indeed, many of us did not even appreciate the fact that minerals were one of six critical nutrients along with vitamins, water, fats, carbohydrates and proteins. This lack of information about minerals prompted me to obtain more research about them in order to give you that information in a way that is understandable and usable.

This book is by no means intended to provide you with a comprehensive list or function of all minerals or describe all the roles they play in disease prevention and management. Instead, my goal is to stimulate an educated discussion about minerals and create a heightened awareness of the important role certain minerals play in preventing and treating various medical issues. We have provided concise and useful information about each of the 14 minerals discussed and explained the most effective ways to obtain testing. Each chapter includes the references used in case you would like to know more about any given topic.

A little bit about my background. I have spent the past three decades as a health care attorney. During this time, I have been lucky enough to work with some of the most talented and dedicated medical professionals, both as their advocate and adversary. I relied on them to give me the knowledge I needed to understand a myriad of health-related issues. In that capacity, I have reviewed well over 50,000 medical records. I learned that had most patients known how to better work with their doctors to improve the effectiveness of treatments, they could have enjoyed much better outcomes. I also learned very early on in my career that being educated about a medical or health issue was one thing, but being able to explain it in such a way that a judge, jury or patient – many of whom had little or no medical background – could understand was quite another task.

Since founding Proactive Health Labs three years ago, I have had the privilege of working closely with three doctors who are committed to educating the public about proactive health care. This team of doctors, Dr. Monya De, Dr. Franz Gliederer and Dr. Pauline J. Jose, are recognized experts in areas as diverse as internal medicine, anti-aging and preventive medicine, occupational medicine, and family medicine. Each brings an unparalleled commitment to helping people make sense of the entire medical and health information available and apply it to get and stay their healthiest.

You can find their biographies at the back of this guide. These doctors have played a critical role in bringing a wide variety of easy-to-understand and easy-to-use information about a broad range of medical and health issues to consumers via www.phlabs.org and especially through the blog series at www.phlabs.org/healthinfo. Topics range from managing nutrition, hypertension and diabetes to using supplements and genomics. With hundreds of topics covered, I am sure you will find many that are both relevant and interesting to you. I invite you to take advantage of this resource.

I hope you find this guide helpful and that you return to it time and time again as you have questions about certain health conditions and about minerals in general. Please feel free to get in touch with us via our website, www.phlabs.org, about any questions you may have about this book, or you can call our toll-free number at 1-855-745-2271. We look forward to hearing from you!

Thanks again and enjoy your healthy life!

Joy Stephenson-Laws
Founder, pH Labs

THE STORY OF MINERALS AND YOU

Every good story hinges on great characters. In this book, you'll be introduced to some of the most underrated characters in history – Minerals.

Like vitamins, minerals are nutrients you get from food that provide nourishment to your body. In fact, there are six types of nutrients that your body cannot live without! They are carbohydrates, fats, proteins, vitamins, minerals and water.

You hear so much about carbs, and how they give you energy and provide fuel for your brain and muscles. You hear so much about protein too, and how you need protein to build strong muscles, hair, skin and nails. Then you have fats. You've been told about the importance of eating healthy fats and avoiding the bad fats, and your doctors monitor your cholesterol levels regularly. Vitamins are, of course, a staple, with many of you taking a multivitamin and choosing vitamin-rich fruits and veggies to stay well. Water is a no-brainer; you've been told about the importance of hydration since elementary school!

On the other hand, much of the information you're told about minerals revolves around the A-listers, calcium and iron. You have heard about calcium since childhood, and how you need calcium for strong bones. Women are encouraged to make sure they eat enough iron because they require more than men. But calcium and iron are only two of the many mineral superstars your body needs to thrive. There are many other critical minerals that you hardly ever hear about such as zinc, copper, selenium, potassium and magnesium, to name a few.

So, how important are minerals? According to two-time Nobel Prize winner Linus Pauling: "You could trace every disease and every ailment to a mineral deficiency." Of course, this statement may be a slight exaggeration to the extent that it fails to account for genetic disorders, but it is fair to say that minerals play a critical role in our health.

In 1618, a farmer in Epsom, England, tried to give his cows water from a well, but they refused to drink it because of its bitter taste. But the farmer noticed the water seemed to heal scratches and rashes. Naturally, the fame of soaking in an Epsom salt (magnesium sulfate) bath began to spread. At this time, magnesium was famous, but without a name.

In the early 19th century, a famous English chemist by the name of Sir Humphry Davy isolated magnesium, along with the minerals potassium, sodium and calcium, using a process called electrolysis (using electric voltage and current to separate minerals). (Fun fact: Though he originally wanted to be a poet, Davy first got his start in the laboratory as a young man inhaling gases in the name of science, including laughing gas.)

Davy's discoveries earned him international recognition and an invitation from Napoleon to visit France. It was there that he was presented with a recently discovered substance that had been isolated from seaweed. Working in his hotel room, Davy studied this new mineral and gave it the name iodine (named after the Greek word for violet because of its purple-colored vapors).

Mineral discoveries like these continued throughout the centuries, coinciding with research on the other classes of nutrients we discussed – proteins, fats and carbohydrates. Vitamin research began to flourish in the early 1900s, leaving minerals to fizzle out of the public spotlight. Vitamins walked the red carpet of the scientific papers, debuting alphabetical names and important health functions. Nobel prize-winning work unveiled vitamins A, B1, B2, B6, B12, C, D, E and K.

In the following chapters, we are going to shine a spotlight on many of these unsung mineral heroes, and explain why you need minerals, how minerals can help you address specific health issues, and how you can be proactive to ensure you are including the right minerals in your diet.

You're writing your own story right now and whether you know it or not, minerals have been a part of your story since the beginning and will be until the end. So, let us share with you the story of minerals throughout these following chapters, so that you can begin the next chapter in your story with knowledge, empowerment and good health.

Enjoy Your Healthy Life!

PART I

MINERALS AND SOME
COMMON HEALTH ISSUES

1

MINERALS AND BLOOD PRESSURE

According to the U.S. Centers for Disease Control and Prevention, nearly a third of Americans - some 90 to 100 million - are diagnosed with high blood pressure. Often called the "silent killer," high blood pressure greatly increases your risk for heart disease and stroke.[1] Persistently elevated blood pressure may not only lead to clogged arteries, heart attacks or strokes, but it may also damage blood vessels, causing kidney impairment, loss of vision, erectile dysfunction, memory loss, fluid in the lungs, angina and peripheral artery disease.[2]

A normal blood pressure reading is generally 120/80 millimeters of mercury or less and an abnormal reading may be 140/90 millimeters of mercury or higher, according to the American Heart Association.[3] While a majority of people are aware they have high blood pressure, very few have their blood pressure sufficiently controlled.[4] Mineral balance may play a huge part in controlling hypertension.

SODIUM (Na) AND POTASSIUM (K)

If you have high blood pressure, your doctor has probably told you to cut back on salty foods. Reducing your sodium intake can help to lower high blood pressure. What your doctor may not have told you is that a good balance of sodium and potassium can also help to reduce blood pressure. Increasing your potassium intake while reducing the sodium intake in your diet may improve hypertension. Increased potassium can offset the adverse health effects of sodium.[5]

Studies show that the sodium/potassium ratio intake should be less than 1. Unfortunately, only 12 percent of the U.S. population has this adequate ratio.[5] The American Heart Association recommends a maximum daily intake of 1,500 mg of sodium, but in reality 99.8 percent of the population consumes much more. The tolerable upper intake level is 2,300 mg daily. Most people actually consume more than 3,000 mg, which is more than twice what is recommended.[6]

Typically, potassium intake is too low or inadequate in the United States. The current daily recommendation for potassium intake is 4,700 mg for adults.[8] A review of 19 clinical studies confirmed that potassium had a positive effect in lowering high blood pressure. Normal or high potassium intake usually does not affect people with normal blood pressure. Specific study findings showed an average reduction of 5.9 mm Hg in systolic blood pressure and 3.4 mm Hg in diastolic blood pressure when increasing potassium in participants' diets. Keeping healthy levels of sodium and potassium may be important for preventing hypertension. Further, doctors may recommend an increase in potassium intake as an alternative to a pharmacological approach to control blood pressure "in uncomplicated essential hypertension."[7]

MAGNESIUM (Mg)

This calming mineral is widely regarded for its muscle-relaxing properties, which may help people with high blood pressure. A review of 22 studies on magnesium and hypertension showed a 3-4 mm Hg reduction of systolic blood pressure and 2-3 mm Hg reduction of diastolic blood pressure.[9] This study used a daily magnesium supplementation of 120-973 mg (average dose 400 mg) over a period of three to 24 weeks. It was noted that the participants' cardiovascular risk was progressively lower among those with higher magnesium dosing. The current recommended daily intake is 360 mg for adult females and 401 mg for adult males, but higher doses may be necessary for people with a deficiency.[10]

REFERENCES

1. Centers for Disease Control and Prevention (CDC). Leading causes of death and numbers of death, by sex, race, and Hispanic origin, United States 1980 and 2014. (2015).

2. American Heart Association: "Why blood pressure matters" Website: http://www.heart.org

3. American Heart Association: "Understanding Blood Pressure" Website: http://www.heart.org

4. Go, A. S. et al. An Effective Approach to High Blood Pressure Control – A Science Advisory From the American Heart Association, the American College of Cardiology, and the Centers for Disease Control and Prevention. Hypertension 63, 878–885 (2014).

5. Bailey, R. L. et al. Estimating Sodium and Potassium Intakes And Their Ratio in the American Diet: Data from the 2011-2012 NHANES. J. Nutr. (2016). doi:10.3945/jn.115.221184

6. Cogswell, M. E. et al. Sodium and potassium intakes among US adults: NHANES 2003–2008. Am. J. Clin. Nutr. 96, 647–657 (2012).

7. Cappuccio, F. P. & MacGregor, G. A. Does potassium supplementation lower blood pressure? A meta-analysis of published trials. J. Hypertens. 9, 465–473 (1991).

8. Appendix 7. Nutritional Goals for Age-Sex Groups Based on Dietary Reference Intakes and Dietary Guidelines Recommendations - 2015-2020 Dietary Guidelines - health. gov. Available at: http://health.gov/dietaryguidelines/2015/ guidelines/appendix-7/. (Accessed: 15th April 2016).

9. Kass, L., Weekes, J. & Carpenter, L. Effect of magnesium supplementation on blood pressure: a meta-analysis. Eur. J. Clin. Nutr. 66, 411–418 (2012).

10. Magnesium Fact sheet. National Institutes of Health. Institute of Dietary Supplements. Website: https://ods.od.nih.gov/ factsheets/Magnesium-HealthProfessional/

2
MINERALS AND WEIGHT MANAGEMENT

Millions of dollars are spent on weight loss every year. Minerals provide some intriguing possibilities in aiding weight loss, yet they get mostly ignored by the press and all those diet books!

MAGNESIUM (Mg)

Let's start with that star mineral, magnesium. In some women, low magnesium is associated with higher rates of obesity and diabetes, although whether it's the low magnesium causing the weight gain or the other way around wasn't examined in that particular study.[1] But there's controversy about this. A study of almost 700 people found that there was no link between being overweight and having low magnesium levels, although low magnesium levels seemed to predict high blood sugar.[2] Studies with rats have shown us that a low magnesium level can slow down growth of lean body mass (muscle and bone building) and promote an increase in body fat![3] This is probably due to the body's need for magnesium in so many different functions. It's no wonder that things slow down and get sluggish without magnesium. Going back to humans, some doctors have posited that magnesium is the key to being overweight but not showing any signs of obesity-related disease – no high blood pressure, diabetes or cholesterol. If you want to read more about this type of patient, search for "MONW" on medical sites. Their reasoning is that overweight people, as discussed above, with low magnesium tend to have high blood sugar.[4] Perhaps the extra muscle (lean body mass) helps to metabolize any extra sugars! No wonder doctors urge diabetic patients to exercise. Perhaps they should be asking them to supplement with magnesium as well.

PHOSPHORUS (P)

Unassuming phosphorus may actually be a key factor in preventing obesity. One theory goes like this: High-carb diets increase insulin release, which creates a reaction that consumes a lot of phosphorus. The phosphorus isn't available to do other reactions in the body, like burn off food. This low metabolism gets mistranslated to the body as "not enough food," which causes us to eat more. Supporting this theory is that high levels of phosphorus in the body are linked with lower body weight.[5] In a study of almost 40,000 women in Korea, phosphorus deficiency correlated with weight gain from oral contraceptives.[6] Even more exciting is a study from Lebanon showing that phosphorus supplements in a small group (63 people) for 12 weeks significantly decreased body weight, BMI, waist circumference and subjective appetite scores. These findings support a promising role of the mineral phosphorus in the prevention and management of obesity, especially abdominal adiposity. The exact mechanisms of action and longer-term effects still need to be elucidated.[7]

IRON (Fe)

There's a lot of research on the link between obesity and iron deficiency. Basically, excess weight seems related to iron deficiency.[8] The *American Journal of Clinical Nutrition* reported on a study involving obese and non-obese women who ate a meal "rigged" to test their iron absorption. In overweight and obese women, iron absorption is two-thirds that in normal-weight women, and the enhancing effect of ascorbic acid (vitamin C) on iron absorption is one-half of that in normal-weight women. This supports the obesity causing the iron deficiency, instead of another explanation like "overweight people don't take vitamins or eat healthy food." The authors recommended that obese women consume extra vitamin C with their iron (or iron-containing food, like meats). Pregnant women who are obese are at extra risk for being iron deficient, and the placenta actually makes more of a certain protein to compensate for this problem.[10] Obese children? Same story. Doctors point out, though, that the common iron test ferritin can be a misleading indicator of iron status in obese people. Because obesity causes low-grade inflammation, and ferritin runs high with high iron or high inflammation, the test can be misleading. A regular "blood iron" test is a better indicator in obese people.[10] Research suggests that the inflammation could cause an increased amount of a protein, hepcidin, leading to iron deficiency.[9]

ZINC (Zn)

What about zinc? Well, a compelling amount of evidence suggests that zinc helps to block the bad effects of obesity in the body. Remember that it has anti-inflammatory properties! In mice, Chinese scientists found that zinc deficiency worsens high-fat diet-induced vascular inflammation and oxidative stress, but the mice who took zinc supplements didn't have these health effects, despite eating the mouse equivalent of donuts and fried chicken.[10] Similarly, mice who ate too much and normally developed kidney damage didn't get it when they took zinc supplements.[13]

Does this mean we should all eat ice cream and down zinc? No! We still don't know if this works as well in humans, and high-fat diets can have other negative consequences (like obesity). What's implied is that obese patients should make sure that their zinc levels are adequate.

REFERENCES

1. Bertinato, J. et al. Lower serum magnesium concentration is associated with diabetes, insulin resistance, and obesity in South Asian and white Canadian women but not men. Food Nutr. Res. 59, 25974 (2015).

2. Guerrero-Romero, F., Flores-García, A., Saldaña-Guerrero, S., Simental-Mendía, L. E. & Rodríguez-Morán, M. Obesity and hypomagnesemia. Eur. J. Intern. Med. (2016). doi:10.1016/j.ejim.2016.06.015

3. Bertinato, J. et al. Moderately Low Magnesium Intake Impairs Growth of Lean Body Mass in Obese-Prone and Obese-Resistant Rats Fed a High-Energy Diet. Nutrients 8, (2016).

4. al, B. J., et. Lower serum magnesium concentration is associated with diabetes, insulin resistance, and obesity in South Asian and white Canadian women but not men. - PubMed - NCBI. Available at: http://www.ncbi.nlm.nih.gov/pubmed/25947295. (Accessed: 1st July 2016).

5. Obeid, O. A. Low phosphorus status might contribute to the onset of obesity. Obes. Rev. Off. J. Int. Assoc. Study Obes. 14, 659–664 (2013).

6. Park, B. & Kim, J. Oral Contraceptive Use, Micronutrient Deficiency, and Obesity among Premenopausal Females in Korea: The Necessity of Dietary Supplements and Food Intake Improvement. PloS One 11, e0158177 (2016).

7. Ayoub, J. J., Samra, M. J. A., Hlais, S. A., Bassil, M. S. & Obeid, O. A. Effect of phosphorus supplementation on weight gain and waist circumference of overweight/obese adults: a randomized clinical trial. Nutr. Diabetes 5, e189 (2015).

8. Zhao, L. et al. Obesity and iron deficiency: a quantitative meta-analysis. Obes. Rev. Off. J. Int. Assoc. Study Obes. 16, 1081–1093 (2015).

9. Nazif, H. K. et al. Study of Serum Hepcidin as a Potential Mediator of the Disrupted Iron Metabolism in Obese Adolescents. Int. J. Health Sci. 9, 172–178 (2015).

10. Chen, J. et al. From the Cover: Zinc Deficiency Worsens and Supplementation Prevents High-Fat Diet Induced Vascular Inflammation, Oxidative Stress, and Pathological Remodeling. Toxicol. Sci. Off. J. Soc. Toxicol. 153, 124–136 (2016).

11. Luo, M. et al. Zinc delays the progression of obesity-related glomerulopathy in mice via down-regulating P38 MAPK-mediated inflammation. Obes. Silver Spring Md 24, 1244–1256 (2016).

3

MINERALS AND DEPRESSION

We all feel unhappy, down or desperate at some point in our lives. These feelings are considered a normal part of life if we usually feel better again after a while. Things are different for people who have depression. With depression, their unhappiness and negative thoughts last longer and overshadow all of their thoughts and actions. Depression can arise without any triggering events or for no apparent reasons. People often feel like they are stuck in a deep pit. They feel cheerless and lack motivation and self-confidence.

Major depression has been cited as the fourth leading cause of disability worldwide. It is anticipated that by 2020, it will be the second leading cause of disability.

Approximately 12 percent of men and 25 percent of women will suffer from depression at some point in their lives. Depression is usually unrecognized because its physical symptoms, such as pain or fatigue, occur with other many other health conditions. People may also be wary of the stigma associated with it and decide not to seek medical help to treat their depression. Certain medical conditions can make it more likely that you will suffer from depression, as does being a member of the "baby boomer" generation (born between 1946 and 1964). Just as with other medical conditions, medications for treating depression may have untoward side effects, prompting studies on depression and how minerals and food could help alleviate symptoms.[1]

MAGNESIUM (Mg)

Several studies have shown an improvement in the severity of symptoms of depression when study participants were given 125-300 mg of magnesium with each meal and at bedtime. Rapid recovery in less than seven days was seen. Symptoms that improved included irritability, insomnia, hopelessness and anxiety. Another study done on treatment-resistant depression, which is estimated to be about 60 percent of individuals suffering from depression, revealed low magnesium brain levels. Low magnesium has also been found in suicidal patients. Early studies dating back to 1921 showed that magnesium works like imipramine, a tricyclic antidepressant, and later studies showed it works for treatment-resistant depression. More studies need to be done to show whether magnesium works as an adjunct to antidepressants or by itself, but many studies are promising enough for magnesium to be recommended if you are suffering from depressive symptoms.[2,3,4,5]

CHROMIUM (Cr)

Many studies have been done to assess the benefit of chromium picolinate in depression. A study of patients with atypical depression showed that 70 percent who took 600 mcg of chromium picolinate had improvement in their symptoms. Another study showed that 65 percent of a group of mostly overweight, depressed people showed improvement in their symptoms when they took the same dose of chromium. Symptoms such as increased appetite, carbohydrate cravings and emotional instability all improved. More studies need to be done, possibly with higher doses of chromium, to find out whether it will improve other symptoms of depression. However, if you are depressed, you might want to discuss with a qualified physician about supplementing your diet with chromium.[7,8,9]

IRON (Fe)

Decreased levels of iron can result in apathy, depression and fatigue. Many women are depressed during their child-bearing years (25-45), and one reason for this could be that women lose iron during menstruation. Iron is also important for oxygenation of the brain and necessary for all its functions. Studies need to be done to find out how common iron deficiency anemia is in patients with depression, and once corrected, to determine which symptoms would be improved. In the meantime, if you are depressed, you should check your iron levels.[10]

SELENIUM (Se)

Depression, as a result of selenium deficiency, has been established in at least five different studies. Depression may be the result of oxidative stress, which is why selenium may be helpful. Selenium has antioxidant properties. Numerous studies done on different populations and age groups suffering from depression showed improvement in mood and anxiety when given selenium. These studies also showed low selenium blood levels in depressed and anxious individuals. Overall mood was also improved when selenium was given to those with depleted levels. [19, 20]

ZINC (Zn)

Zinc is a trace element that is essential to the human body. It is involved in over 300 reactions in the body and is abundant in the brain. Many clinical studies have been done to determine the relationship between zinc and depression. Zinc levels are generally low in those with major depression. Zinc supplementation along with antidepressant therapy has been studied and has shown benefits. These studies also showed improvement in depressive symptoms among people whom antidepressants initially didn't help, indicating the real potential for zinc to help augment previously resistant medications. While it is clear that zinc can help in depression by itself or as an adjunct to antidepressants and other vitamins, more research still needs to be done in this area.[9,11,12]

COPPER (Cu)

Copper is important in depression because it is a component of the enzymes that metabolize the brain chemicals that help you respond to stress, feel happy and be alert. These enzymes, and the associated chemicals, are responsible for the causes and treatment of anxiety and depression. Several studies have been done on copper levels and depression, and there is an association between high levels of copper and depression. Antidepressant treatment was also found to reduce copper levels in those tested.[13,14,15]

MANGANESE (Mn)

Manganese is a large component of dismutase (SOD) and was found to be low in the depressive episode of bipolar patients compared to controls. Treatment with the antidepressant fluoxetine increased the level of this enzyme. SOD is important in anti-oxidation and many studies have established that depression is an oxidative process, or can be caused by lack of antioxidants. Chronic exposure to manganese may cause depression. When feeling blue, you might want to check your blood mineral level, especially manganese.[14,16,17]

CALCIUM (Ca)

There is no clear relationship between calcium and depression. Some studies found low calcium in depressed patients and others found elevated levels. However, you cannot ignore calcium's role because it affects the levels of magnesium in the body. Magnesium is important in depression, and if your calcium is too high, it may cause your magnesium to be low, which may make your depressive symptoms harder to treat.

REFERENCES

1. Feldman, M. & Christensen. Behavioral medicine : a guide for clinical practice. Chapter 25 : Depression. (McGraw-Hill, 2014).

2. Eby, G. A. & Eby, K. L. Rapid recovery from major depression using magnesium treatment. Med. Hypotheses 67, 362–370 (2006).

3. Lakhan, S. E. & Vieira, K. F. Nutritional therapies for mental disorders. Nutr. J. 7, 2 (2008).

4. Eby, G. A. & Eby, K. L. Magnesium for treatment-resistant depression: a review and hypothesis. Med. Hypotheses 74, 649–660 (2010).

5. Banki, C. M., Vojnik, M., Papp, Z., Balla, K. Z. & Arató, M. Cerebrospinal fluid magnesium and calcium related to amine metabolites, diagnosis, and suicide attempts. Biol. Psychiatry 20, 163–171 (1985).

6. Serefko, A. et al. Magnesium in depression. Pharmacol. Rep. PR 65, 547–554 (2013).

7. Davidson, J. R. T., Abraham, K., Connor, K. M. & McLeod, M. N. Effectiveness of chromium in atypical depression: a placebo-controlled trial. Biol. Psychiatry 53, 261–264 (2003).

8. Docherty, J. P., Sack, D. A., Roffman, M., Finch, M. & Komorowski, J. R. A double-blind, placebo-controlled, exploratory trial of chromium picolinate in atypical depression: effect on carbohydrate craving. J. Psychiatr. Pract. 11, 302–314 (2005).

9. Rao, T. S. S., Asha, M. R., Ramesh, B. N. & Rao, K. S. J. Understanding nutrition, depression and mental illnesses. Indian J. Psychiatry 50, 77–82 (2008).

10. Bourre, J. M. Effects of nutrients (in food) on the structure and function of the nervous system: update on dietary requirements for brain. Part 1: micronutrients. J. Nutr. Health Aging 10, 377–385 (2006).

11. Lai, J. et al. The efficacy of zinc supplementation in depression: systematic review of – controlled trials. J. Affect. Disord. 136, e31–39 (2012).

12. Nowak, G., Szewczyk, B. & Pilc, A. Zinc and depression. An update. Pharmacol. Rep. PR 57, 713–718 (2005).

13. Młyniec, K. et al. Essential elements in depression and anxiety. Part II. Pharmacol. Rep. PR 67, 187–194 (2015).

14. Gosney, M. A., Hammond, M. F., Shenkin, A. & Allsup, S. Effect of micronutrient supplementation on mood in nursing home residents. Gerontology 54, 292–299 (2008).

15. Narang, R. L., Gupta, K. R., Narang, A. P. & Singh, R. Levels of copper and zinc in depression. Indian J. Physiol. Pharmacol. 35, 272–274 (1991).

16. Gałecki, P., Szemraj, J., Bieńkiewicz, M., Florkowski, A. & Gałecka, E. Lipid peroxidation and antioxidant protection in patients during acute depressive episodes and in remission after fluoxetine treatment. Pharmacol. Rep. PR 61, 436–447 (2009).

17. Bowler, R. M., Mergler, D., Sassine, M. P., Larribe, F. & Hudnell, K. Neuropsychiatric effects of manganese on mood. Neurotoxicology 20, 367–378 (1999).

18. Shor-Posner, G. et al. Psychological burden in the era of HAART: impact of selenium therapy. Int. J. Psychiatry Med. 33, 55–69 (2003)/

19. Pasco, J. A. et al. Dietary selenium and major depression: a nested case-control study. Complement. Ther. Med. 20, 119–123 (2012).

20. Benton, D. Selenium intake, mood and other aspects of psychological functioning. Nutr. Neurosci. 5, 363–374 (2002).

4

MINERALS AND PRESCRIPTION DRUGS

Did you know that common medications may deplete your body of the key minerals you need to be your healthiest? Prescription drugs may improve your health, but they all have side effects. Any effect of a drug that is in addition to its intended effect, is considered a side effect, and some of these side effects may involve the depletion or increase of certain minerals. A deficiency in magnesium, potassium, sodium, calcium, iron or zinc may be responsible for some of your side effects.

If you take prescription drugs, you may need to get a micronutrient test and supplement specific minerals under the direction of a physician to get back to feeling like yourself. Here are some of the "mineral-depleters" you need to be aware of:

DIURETICS

Diuretics reduce swelling and high blood pressure due to fluid overload. They are sometimes referred to as "water pills" because they increase the amount of water released from your body. The increased water loss may also cause the loss of essential minerals in the body. If these mineral deficits are not addressed, adverse health outcomes, such as fatigue and a myriad of other symptoms, may occur.

Sodium (Na), Potassium (K), Magnesium (Mg), Zinc (Zn) & Calcium (Ca)

Thiazide diuretics (such as hydrochlorothiazide and chlorthalidone) are commonly used in primary care practice to treat high blood pressure.[1] They often cause losses of sodium, potassium, magnesium, zinc and calcium. What happens is they inhibit your body's ability to reabsorb these minerals in the kidneys, so they end up getting excreted out via urine.[2] Since many people with high blood pressure need to reduce their sodium,[3] this is frequently a desirable effect. On the other hand, with prolonged use, it can cause excess sodium depletion. So levels need to be monitored.

Low potassium and magnesium from extended use of diuretics can increase blood pressure. The reverse is also true; addition of potassium supplements can help to lower blood pressure.[4,5] Some diuretics can cause zinc loss and sexual dysfunction, and some studies indicate that zinc treatment can help with sexual dysfunction.[6,8] Loop diuretics, such as furosemide (Lasix), cause excess calcium loss.[9]

- Diuretics can cause mineral deficiencies. They can cause loss of potassium, magnesium, zinc, calcium or even sodium to unhealthful levels.
- When taking diuretics, mineral levels should be checked with your doctor.
- Deficits are correctable with supplements and mineral-rich foods.[10]

ANTACIDS, PROTON PUMP INHIBITORS, H$_2$ BLOCKERS

Antacids, proton pump inhibitors and H$_2$ blockers are used to combat reflux disease (GERD) and heartburn and to prevent gastric ulcers. While prescription drugs can be quite effective at reducing the acidity,

acidity serves several purposes. It helps absorb certain nutrients, helps to digest foods better, and can also kill bacteria, viruses or other infectious diseases.[11]

Minerals that require an acidic environment to work well may not be effective when we take these drugs.[11,12,13]

Zinc (Zn) and Calcium (Ca)

Zinc absorption works better in an acidic environment, and a study showed decreased zinc absorption after the administration of an H_2 blocker – Tagamet (cimetidine). Generally, these medications should be used for a limited time period.[13] Talk to your doctor if you feel you can't get off these medications. Other newer antacids (proton pump inhibitors, PPIs) are associated with less calcium absorption which may cause brittle bones.[13]

ANTIHYPERTENSIVES & HEART MEDICATIONS

Antihypertensives are blood pressure medications that may also affect your mineral balance.

Zinc (Zn) and Potassium (K)

Patients with heart failure taking ACE inhibitors may have lower zinc levels and higher zinc urinary excretion.[35,36] Calcium channel blockers, such as nifedipine, verapamil or diltiazem, interfere with potassium, causing an increase in potassium inside your cells and a decrease in potassium in your blood, raising the risk of high blood pressure and irregular heart rhythm.[37]

Digoxin

Digoxin, a heart failure medication, has special importance since its mineral depletions of potassium and magnesium increase the likelihood of life-threatening heart arrhythmias.[38] That's why doctors have to carefully measure the levels of digoxin and minerals in the blood of heart patients who take it.

ANTIBIOTICS

Antibiotics are drugs used to treat a variety of infections. There are different types of antibiotics and their presence in your body may affect the absorption of certain minerals.

Calcium (Ca), Iron (Fe) & Potassium (K)

One type of antibiotics – fluoroquinolones such as levofloxacin, ciprofloxacin or moxifloxacin – can interact with calcium and iron, reducing available calcium and iron for your body to use.[14]

Another type of antibiotic, trimethoprim, may interfere with your body's ability to get rid of extra potassium, contributing to high potassium levels.[16] Signs of this may include weakness and fatigue, muscle cramps and pain, worsening diabetes, palpitations and psychiatric symptoms (like psychosis, delirium, hallucinations or depression).

Tetracyclines, penicillins, amphotericin B and aminoglycosides can induce kidney dysfunction.[18] Another one to watch: Gentamicin causes immediate calcium and magnesium loss by impairing your kidney function. You will likely need supplements if on this antibiotic for a prolonged period. Monitoring electrolyte levels was endorsed especially with longer-term antibiotic therapy.[20,19]

OVER-THE-COUNTER DRUGS (OTC)

Even though OTC medications do not need a doctor's prescription, they can have side effects and interactions. Commonly used OTC medications such as ibuprofen (Advil, Motrin) can also cause kidney impairment and mineral losses or inability to excrete minerals.[21]

ANTIEPILEPTICS

Anticonvulsant medications are used to treat patients for seizures, pain syndromes and other conditions. These medications are linked to a 20-40 percent increased osteoporosis risk. Why? Antiepileptics cause extra enzyme activity in the liver. This leads to accelerated churning of vitamin D, and insufficient vitamin D is linked to mineral depletion in bones.[25] In white populations over 50 years of age, 50 percent of women and 20 percent of men will have brittle bones over the course of their remaining life span.[25] Vitamin D testing is one of the best ways to determine if this side effect is occurring.

HORMONE THERAPY

Hormone therapy may influence minerals such as magnesium and bone mineral density positively, but at different doses of hormones (like with birth control pills or the non-estrogen Depo-Provera), there can be bone loss.[26,30] Women who take menopausal hormone therapy also have better copper and zinc levels.[31] Studies found that birth control pill users had lower magnesium,[33,34] calcium and phosphorus [33] than those who did not.

REFERENCES

1. Clayton, J. A. & Rodgers, S. Thiazide diuretic prescription and electrolyte abnormalities in primary care. Br. J. Clin. Pharmacol. 61, 87–95 (2006).

2. Reyes, A. J. Effects of diuretics on outputs and flows of urine and urinary solutes in healthy subjects. Drugs 41 Suppl 3, 35–59 (1991).

3. Yang, Q. & Liu, T. Sodium and potassium intake and mortality among US adults: prospective data from the Third National Health and Nutrition Examination Survey. Arch. Intern. Med. 171, 1183–1191 (2011).

4. Cappuccio, F. P. & MacGregor, G. A. Does potassium supplementation lower blood pressure? A meta-analysis of published trials. J. Hypertens. 9, 465–473 (1991).

5. Pak, C. Y. Correction of thiazide-induced hypomagnesemia by potassium-magnesium citrate from review of prior trials. Clin. Nephrol. 54, 271–275 (2000).

6. Reyes, A. J., Olhaberry, J. V., Leary, W. P., Lockett, C. J. & van der Byl, K. Urinary zinc excretion, diuretics, zinc deficiency and some side-effects of diuretics. South Afr. Med. J. Suid-Afr. Tydskr. Vir Geneeskd. 64, 936–941 (1983).

7. Chiba, M. et al. Diuretics aggravate zinc deficiency in patients with liver cirrhosis by increasing zinc excretion in urine. Hepatol. Res. Off. J. Jpn. Soc. Hepatol. 43, 365–373 (2013).

8. Khedun, S. M., Naicker, T. & Maharaj, B. Zinc, hydrochlorothiazide and sexual dysfunction. Cent. Afr. J. Med. 41, 312–315 (1995).

9. Vasco, R. F. V., Moyses, R. M. A., Zatz, R. & Elias, R. M. Furosemide Increases the Risk of Hyperparathyroidism in Chronic Kidney Disease. Am. J. Nephrol. 43, 421–430 (2016).

10. Ruml, L. A., Gonzalez, G., Taylor, R., Wuermser, L. A. & Pak, C. Y. Effect of varying doses of potassium-magnesium citrate on thiazide-induced hypokalemia and magnesium loss. Am. J. Ther. 6, 45–50 (1999).

11. Abramowitz, J. et al. Adverse Event Reporting for Proton Pump Inhibitor Therapy: An Overview of Systematic Reviews. Otolaryngol. – Head Neck Surg. Off. J. Am. Acad. Otolaryngol.- Head Neck Surg. (2016). doi:10.1177/0194599816648298

12. Sturniolo, G. C. et al. Inhibition of gastric acid secretion reduces zinc absorption in man. J. Am. Coll. Nutr. 10, 372–375 (1991).

13. Murphy, C. E. et al. Frequency of inappropriate continuation of acid suppressive therapy after discharge in patients who began therapy in the surgical intensive care unit. Pharmacotherapy 28, 968–976 (2008).

14. Deppermann, K. M. & Lode, H. Fluoroquinolones: interaction profile during enteral absorption. Drugs 45 Suppl 3, 65–72 (1993).

15. Stass, H. & Kubitza, D. Effects of iron supplements on the oral bioavailability of moxifloxacin, a novel 8-methoxyfluoroquinolone, in humans. Clin. Pharmacokinet. 40 Suppl 1, 57–62 (2001).

16. Ben Salem, C., Badreddine, A., Fathallah, N., Slim, R. & Hmouda, H. Drug-induced hyperkalemia. Drug Saf. 37, 677–692 (2014).

17. Zaki, S. A. & Lad, V. Piperacillin-tazobactam-induced hypokalemia and metabolic alkalosis. Indian J. Pharmacol. 43, 609–610 (2011).

18. Zietse, R., Zoutendijk, R. & Hoorn, E. J. Fluid, electrolyte and acid-base disorders associated with antibiotic therapy. Nat. Rev. Nephrol. 5, 193–202 (2009).

19. Elliott, C., Newman, N. & Madan, A. Gentamicin effects on urinary electrolyte excretion in healthy subjects. Clin. Pharmacol. Ther. 67, 16–21 (2000).

20. Kasama, R. & Sorbello, A. Renal and electrolyte complications associated with antibiotic therapy. Am. Fam. Physician 53, 227–232 (1996).

21. Whelton, A. Renal effects of over-the-counter analgesics. J. Clin. Pharmacol. 35, 454–463 (1995).

22. Freytag, A. et al. [Use and potential risks of over-the-counter analgesics]. Schmerz Berl. Ger. 28, 175–182 (2014).

23. Schmiedl, S. et al. Self-medication with over-the-counter and prescribed drugs causing adverse-drug-reaction-related hospital admissions: results of a prospective, long-term multicentre study. Drug Saf. 37, 225–235 (2014).

24. Qato, D. M. et al. Use of Prescription and Over-the-counter Medications and Dietary Supplements Among Older Adults in the United States. JAMA J. Am. Med. Assoc. 300, 2867–2878 (2008).

25. Lee, R. H., Lyles, K. W. & Colón-Emeric, C. A Review of the Effect of Anticonvulsant Medications on Bone Mineral Density and Fracture Risk. Am. J. Geriatr. Pharmacother. 8, 34–46 (2010).

26. Jurczak, A. et al. Effect of menopausal hormone therapy on the levels of magnesium, zinc, lead and cadmium in post-menopausal women. Ann. Agric. Environ. Med. AAEM 20, 147–151 (2013).

27. Bureau, I. et al. Trace mineral status in post menopausal women: impact of hormonal replacement therapy. J. Trace Elem. Med. Biol. Organ Soc. Miner. Trace Elem. GMS 16, 9–13 (2002).

28. Zofková, I. & Kancheva, R. L. Effect of estrogen status on bone regulating hormones. Bone 19, 227–232 (1996).

29. Sahota, O., Mundey, M. K., San, P., Godber, I. M. & Hosking, D. J. Vitamin D insufficiency and the blunted PTH response in established osteoporosis: the role of magnesium deficiency. Osteoporos. Int. J. Establ. Result Coop. Eur. Found. Osteoporos. Natl. Osteoporos. Found. USA 17, 1013–1021 (2006).

30. Tolaymat, L. L. & Kaunitz, A. M. Use of hormonal contraception in adolescents: skeletal health issues. Curr. Opin. Obstet. Gynecol. 21, 396–401 (2009).

31. Bureau, I. et al. Trace mineral status in post menopausal women: impact of hormonal replacement therapy. J. Trace Elem. Med. Biol. Organ Soc. Miner. Trace Elem. GMS 16, 9–13 (2002).

32. Blasig, S. et al. Positive correlation of thyroid hormones and serum copper in children with congenital hypothyroidism. J. Trace Elem. Med. Biol. Organ Soc. Miner. Trace Elem. GMS (2016). doi:10.1016/j.jtemb.2016.05.007

33. Hameed, A. et al. Effect of oral and injectable contraceptives on serum calcium, magnesium and phosphorus in women. J. Ayub Med. Coll. Abbottabad JAMC 13, 24–25 (2001).

34. Olatunbosun, D. A., Adeniyi, F. A. & Adadevoh, B. K. Effect of oral contraceptives on Serum magnesium levels. Int. J. Fertil. 19, 224–226 (1974).

35. Trasobares, E. et al. Effects of angiotensin-converting enzyme inhibitors (ACE i) on zinc metabolism in patients with heart failure. J. Trace Elem. Med. Biol. Organ Soc. Miner. Trace Elem. GMS 21 Suppl 1, 53–55 (2007).

36. Cohen, N. & Golik, A. Zinc balance and medications commonly used in the management of heart failure. Heart Fail. Rev. 11, 19–24 (2006).

37. Li, X.-T., Li, X.-Q., Hu, X.-M. & Qiu, X.-Y. The Inhibitory Effects of Ca2+ Channel Blocker Nifedipine on Rat Kv2.1 Potassium Channels. PLoS ONE 10, (2015).

38. Iezhitsa, I. N. Potassium and magnesium depletions in congestive heart failure – pathophysiology, consequences and replenishment. Clin. Calcium 15, 123–133 (2005).

Other useful article: A Practical Guide to Avoiding Drug-Induced Nutrient Depletion. Hyla Cass, MD

5

MINERALS AND THE BRAIN

PARKINSON'S DISEASE

Parkinson's disease is a disorder of the brain that results in a stiff gait, blank facial expression and involuntary shaking. In Parkinson's patients, zinc and iron are increased and copper is decreased in an area of the midbrain called the substantia nigra. One Japanese study sought to match this information with dietary patterns in Parkinson's patients, in order to see if perhaps zinc and iron consumption caused the disease. In fact, based on patient's recollection of dietary habits, higher consumption of iron, magnesium, and zinc appeared to protect against Parkinson's, while copper consumption didn't really matter. Of course, it's possible that what people remembered eating wasn't actually that accurate, especially since a study of blood levels of minerals in Parkinson's patients begged to differ. In that study, Parkinson's patients had lower copper levels than healthy people![1] Clearly, the science is still being worked out on this issue.

Manganese (Mn)

Manganism is a condition of Parkinson's-like symptoms caused by too much manganese in the body or by a problem in the body's ability to get rid of extra manganese. The extra mineral settles in a part of the brain that controls movements and exerts toxic effects on neurotransmitters like dopamine, hence the tremors, rigidity, and shakes. Don't worry about eating too many nuts and getting shaky, though; manganism usually happens in people who work around manganese in industrial settings.[2]

ALZHEIMER'S DISEASE

Alzheimer's disease is a form of dementia that occurs when the brain develops visible changes like protein deposits and "neurofibrillary tangles." Patients decline over a number of years, losing the ability to recognize faces and communicate.

Selenium (Se)

Selenium, an antioxidant, has shown growing evidence for protection against Alzheimer's disease. In rats, one study showed that treatment with selenium prevented some of the negative effects of aluminum chloride poisoning, which results in rat Alzheimer's disease. (That's why so many doctors are advocating that you use aluminum-free deodorant!) The aluminum promoted oxidative stress and free radicals, impairing memory in the rats, but selenium-treated rats were spared this effect.[3] What about humans? So far, no one has proven that you can treat Alzheimer's with selenium. However, individuals who carry genetic markers for the disease have hope; scientists are fairly certain that good selenium levels have a preventive effect for Alzheimer's![4]

Chromium (Cr)

Alzheimer's is often called "type 3 diabetes," because it seems closely linked to mis-regulated blood sugar. Since we know chromium helps to regulate blood sugar, it's no surprise that chromium supplements help improve test scores in these patients and cause the brain to light up more on a functional MRI, a type of MRI that demonstrates where brain activity is actually happening.[5]

Copper (Cu)

Copper is another mineral implicated in Alzheimer's disease. What exactly happens with copper in the body is still a bit confusing to researchers. While copper supplementation seems to prevent early death in Alzheimer's rats and seems to decrease levels of the culprit beta-amyloid protein that ends up invading the brain in this disease, the answer isn't as simple as just giving everyone more copper. The current thought is that copper needs to be delicately balanced in the body, like sodium and potassium, and that gene mutations you find in people with Alzheimer's could be messing up how the body handles copper.[6,7] Some are even advocating a low-copper diet to prevent Alzheimer's, figuring that the excessive copper many people get in tap water is causing some of this copper dysfunction![8]

MINERALS AND YOUR BRAIN POWER

Can minerals actually make you smarter? This is an interesting area of study. As we know, it's easy to end up with too much of a good thing. We'll show you how mineral deficiencies, once corrected, can make a measurable difference when scientists test animals, children, and adults on cognitive tasks and memory.

Selenium (Se)

Selenium is a big player in brainpower. We've known for a long time that selenium deficiency equals brain development problems in animals, but the research on humans in the 2010s is backing that up as well. When pregnant women in one study were deficient in selenium, their kids ended up being language-delayed and had problems with mental development. Girls were especially affected, for unknown reasons.[9] Another group showed that cognitive function slides down in parallel with decreasing blood selenium levels in older adults.[10]

Excess Copper (Cu)

Mineral excesses can, unfortunately, decrease brain power. Take a study of Chinese adolescents; in the group of kids that had the highest levels of copper in the blood, working memory (important for decision-making) was diminished in boys. Apparently, some kids had extra copper just from their diets (possibly more organ meats or shellfish, though that wasn't measured) or from the pipes providing their drinking water. We do know that boys are more sensitive to copper excess, though we don't know why.[11]

Excess Manganese (Mn) and Chromium (Cr)

Manganese and chromium, in excess amounts, have been linked to cognitive problems in a Mexico City study of young people (the high levels were thought to be due to bad air pollution).[12]

Excess Sodium (Na)

As with so many other bodily functions, sodium and potassium need to be balanced for optimal brain power. In heart failure patients, who often have imbalanced sodium and potassium, due to eating more salt than their bodies can handle, performance on cognitive tests can be impaired.[13]

BRAIN TRAUMA

Because of the high number of brain injuries (concussions and worse) in young people and military personnel, scientists are avidly researching this type of trauma. Animal experiments suggest that magnesium treatment could be good for trauma.[14] The injury disrupts the delicate sodium/potassium balance, meaning that treatments focusing on this area could be useful in these injuries.[15] That's not all; body-wide severe low potassium occurs in hospitalized brain injury patients, often leading to too-low phosphorus and excessively high sodium.[16]

AUTISM

Autism, a brain disorder diagnosed in childhood by its characteristic repetitive movements and behaviors and impaired social functioning, is an area of intense interest for scientists. The apparent epidemic among children in the last few decades, seemingly out of nowhere, has led to a lot of studies on the possible roles minerals could be playing in autism.

Doctors now think that autism arises from a combination of unlucky genes and environmental factors. These environmental factors could include deficiencies of zinc and magnesium and high levels of cadmium, lead, mercury, and arsenic, according to environmental scientists.[17]

A study of 44 autistic kids and 61 healthy children's hair revealed that the autistic kids had higher hair levels of molybdenum, lithium and selenium. Does this mean that pregnant women shouldn't consume molybdenum or selenium? No! There's a lot of possibilities here — perhaps the extra minerals aren't actually causing anything bad; perhaps they are a result of the metabolism of an autistic child's body and not the cause of medical symptoms. Of course, doctors agree that excessive vitamin and mineral supplementation is not advisable in pregnancy, or any other time. If you're hitting 10,000 times the recommended daily allowance of anything, it is time to cut back!

Nutrition researchers agree. A 2015 study concluded that autistic children are often supplemented to the point of excessive levels of certain nutrients, including zinc, copper, and manganese, while sadly ending up with persistent calcium and vitamin D deficiencies in spite of multivitamins.[18] The popular gluten-free, casein-free diet, used by many parents, may be why parents are rushing to supplement, figuring that the missing dairy and wheat is leading to vitamin deficiencies, but kids may actually be getting adequate amounts of these nutrients from the foods they do eat.

Another interesting point the hair study made is that autistic children who had been on "chelation" protocols (diets or treatments meant to trap metals like lead and get them out of the body), didn't have any lower levels than the non-chelating kids. So, this may not be the best investment for a family treating an autistic child.[19]

ADHD

Attention deficit hyperactivity disorder, found in children and adults, is a disorder of executive functioning in the brain. Patients may have hyperactivity, restlessness, inattention, or impulsivity. A demand for answers to this condition has fueled interest in mineral deficiencies that could lead to hyperactivity in children or make it worse.

Zinc and magnesium have popularly been used to treat ADHD. Zinc, for example, works to funnel dopamine around the body, and dopamine helps with focus and motivation.[20] Zinc levels are fairly low in the disease. One small study compared levels of zinc, magnesium, and copper in ADHD children to healthy children. Levels of zinc and magnesium were low in the ADHD kids, but copper levels were normal.[21] However, a systematic review (study of studies) didn't find any tangible benefit with zinc treatment in any of the studies they considered "well-run."

As far as magnesium goes, there hasn't been a solid study establishing that it helps. However, magnesium can always be tried to improve sleep in a child with ADHD, and certainly in a child with a documented magnesium deficiency.[22]

More studies are needed to determine if mineral deficiencies in neurological disorders are the cause of the disorder or an effect of having the rogue genes that cause the disorder. Either way, a child or adult with ADHD could benefit from testing mineral levels and correcting any deficiencies.

REFERENCES

1. Younes-Mhenni, S. & Aissi, M. Serum copper, zinc and selenium levels in Tunisian patients with Parkinson's disease. Tunis. Médicale 91, 402–405 (2013).

2. Kwakye, G. F., Paoliello, M. M. B., Mukhopadhyay, S., Bowman, A. B. & Aschner, M. Manganese-Induced Parkinsonism and Parkinson's Disease: Shared and Distinguishable Features. Int. J. Environ. Res. Public. Health 12, 7519–7540 (2015).

3. Lakshmi, B. V. S. & Sudhakar, M. Protective effect of selenium against aluminum chloride-induced Alzheimer's disease: behavioral and biochemical alterations in rats. Biol. Trace Elem. Res. 165, 67–74 (2015).

4. Loef, M., Schrauzer, G. N. & Walach, H. Selenium and Alzheimer's disease: a systematic review. J. Alzheimers Dis. JAD 26, 81–104 (2011).

5. Krikorian, R., Eliassen, J. C., Boespflug, E. L., Nash, T. A. & Shidler, M. D. Improved cognitive-cerebral function in older adults with chromium supplementation. Nutr. Neurosci. 13, 116–122 (2010).

6. Kessler, H. & Pajonk, F.-G. Effect of copper intake on CSF parameters in patients with mild Alzheimer's disease: a pilot phase 2 clinical trial. J. Neural Transm. Vienna Austria 1996 115, 1651–1659 (2008).

7. Pal, A., Siotto, M., Prasad, R. & Squitti, R. Towards a unified vision of copper involvement in Alzheimer's disease: a review connecting basic, experimental, and clinical research. J. Alzheimers Dis. JAD 44, 343–354 (2015).

8. Squitti, R., Siotto, M. & Polimanti, R. Low-copper diet as a preventive strategy for Alzheimer's disease. Neurobiol. Aging 35 Suppl 2, S40-50 (2014).

9. Skröder, H. M. et al. Selenium status in pregnancy influences children's cognitive function at 1.5 years of age. Clin. Nutr. Edinb. Scotl. 34, 923–930 (2015).

10. Rita Cardoso, B., Silva Bandeira, V., Jacob-Filho, W. & Franciscato Cozzolino, S. M. Selenium status in elderly: relation to cognitive decline. J. Trace Elem. Med. Biol. Organ Soc. Miner. Trace Elem. GMS 28, 422–426 (2014).

11. Zhou, G. et al. Association between Serum Copper Status and Working Memory in Schoolchildren. Nutrients 7, 7185–7196 (2015).

12. Calderón-Garcidueñas, L. et al. The impact of environmental metals in young urbanites' brains. Exp. Toxicol. Pathol. Off. J. Ges. Für Toxikol. Pathol. 65, 503–511 (2013).

13. Hwang, S. Y. & Kim, J. An examination of the association of cognitive functioning, adherence to sodium restriction and Na/K ratios in Korean heart failure patients. J. Clin. Nurs. 25, 1766–1776 (2016).

14. Curtis, L. & Epstein, P. Nutritional treatment for acute and chronic traumatic brain injury patients. J. Neurosurg. Sci. 58, 151–160 (2014).

15. Ha, Y., Jeong, J. A., Kim, Y. & Churchill, D. G. Sodium and Potassium Relating to Parkinson's Disease and Traumatic Brain Injury. Met. Ions Life Sci. 16, 585–601 (2016).

16. Wu, X. et al. Prevalence of severe hypokalaemia in patients with traumatic brain injury. Injury 46, 35–41 (2015).

17. De Palma, G., Catalani, S., Franco, A., Brighenti, M. & Apostoli, P. Lack of correlation between metallic elements analyzed in hair by ICP-MS and autism. J. Autism Dev. Disord. 42, 342–353 (2012).

18. Stewart, P. A. et al. Dietary Supplementation in Children with Autism Spectrum Disorders: Common, Insufficient, and Excessive. J. Acad. Nutr. Diet. 115, 1237–1248 (2015).

19. Lepping, P. & Huber, M. Role of zinc in the pathogenesis of attention-deficit hyperactivity disorder: implications for research and treatment. CNS Drugs 24, 721–728 (2010).

20. Mahmoud, M. M., El-Mazary, A.-A. M., Maher, R. M. & Saber, M. M. Zinc, ferritin, magnesium and copper in a group of Egyptian children with attention deficit hyperactivity disorder. Ital. J. Pediatr. 37, 60 (2011).

21. Ghanizadeh, A. & Berk, M. Zinc for treating of children and adolescents with attention-deficit hyperactivity disorder: a systematic review of randomized controlled clinical trials. Eur. J. Clin. Nutr. 67, 122–124 (2013).

22. Ghanizadeh, A. A systematic review of magnesium therapy for treating attention deficit hyperactivity disorder. Arch. Iran. Med. 16, 412–417 (2013).

6

MINERALS AND THE HEART

Your heart is a muscle with electrical activity constantly running through it. That's what keeps you alive! Minerals play a big role in whether the right electrical impulses fire with the right strength and at the right times. Mineral balance is a key part of good heart health.

MAGNESIUM (Mg) AND CALCIUM (Ca)

Magnesium's importance for the heart can't be overstated. Let's take a quick tour of all the ways this mineral protects your heart. But, we'll also talk about it in the context of its "opposite," calcium.

Magnesium influences heart muscle energy production, keeps calcium levels balanced, loosens up tight blood vessels, reduces inflammation, and keeps all that electrical activity we talked about behaving properly. You can think of calcium as "Fire" and magnesium as "Hold your fire!" in the heart. When calcium causes contraction, squeezing, and high blood pressure, magnesium is a relaxer. But that doesn't mean we should avoid calcium and take a ton of magnesium. An overly high magnesium level can cause cardiac arrest. Low magnesium, on the other hand, may result in atherosclerosis (plaque formation in the arteries), calcifications (calcium deposits in the blood vessels), or blood clots. All of these increase the risk of heart attack.[1] In fact, one study demonstrated that patients who lived in areas with more magnesium in the drinking water had lower rates of heart disease![2] Low magnesium has actually been found to lead to worse outcomes in patients with heart disease, and to higher risk of irregular heartbeat.[3] Now, cardiologists are treating heart disease with magnesium. So, heart attack patients get a daily magnesium (the dose depends on the magnesium formulation), and arrhythmia patients get IV magnesium. Integrative doctors are often adding magnesium to the regimens of patients who can't quite get their blood pressures under control with the regular drugs. Soon, a magnesium level check may be part of the annual physical for people 50 and over.

As for calcium, just as with magnesium, very high or very low levels can cause a cardiac emergency. In a high-calcium state, cardiac conduction abnormalities and arrhythmias can occur (problems with the heart's electrical impulses and rhythm). Your body regulates calcium tightly, dumping what it doesn't need and recruiting calcium from bones when it needs more, so it usually takes a serious medical problem to cause calcium levels to rise about 15 mg/dL (enough to cause cardiac arrest). Cancer, parathyroid disease and kidney disease are some of the causes of high calcium (usually not drinking too much milk!). Low calcium can cause electrical abnormalities as well. This condition requires there to be something really wrong with the body, like severe pneumonia or significant burns.

Calcification or calcium deposits in the heart's arteries (coronaries) are a hot topic in medical research. The reason is that doctors want to know whether taking too many calcium supplements can actually increase risk for heart disease; can extra calcium just get dumped into the arteries and harden them?[4] A review of studies, rather, shows that phosphorus from food preservatives and sodas might actually cause calcification, and that free radicals could as well. Preventers of calcification include: having a high folate level, consuming resveratrol from red wine and antioxidant catechins in green tea, avoiding sugar and trans fats, and consuming magnesium and vitamin K.[5]

SODIUM (Na) AND POTASSIUM (K)

Sodium can influence the actual size of the heart, believe it or not. A large heart sounds great, but when an international group of scientists studied people with high blood pressure, those who recalled consuming a lot of sodium in their diets had "stretched," enlarged heart chambers.[6] This enlargement ages the heart and makes the heart function less well in pumping blood.

How good is your response to stress? Sodium can influence a measure of stress known as heart rate variability. Heart rate variability is a good thing; you want your heart to be toned like any other muscle, able to relax and beat slowly in times of low stress and able to rev up when you are in need of quick movements or quick thinking. In people with both too-low and too-high dietary sodium intake, heart rate variability was disrupted in one study.[7]

Too much potassium can be a culprit too. Many emergencies in the ER are due to high potassium levels, usually from a combination of eating too much potassium-containing food and one of many common medications that lower blood pressure (look for the ones that end in –il or –tan in particular). What happens is potassium disrupts the electrical activity of the heart—this can lead to a fatal arrhythmia, or irregular heartbeat. One study of patients showed that heart conduction was most disrupted when people who were either too thin or too heavy consumed a lot of potassium.[3] All of this shows us that our bodies really like to be in balance. Not too much (food or potassium) and not too little. This is why extreme or restrictive diets are never a good idea.

REFERENCES

1. de Baaij, J. H. F., Hoenderop, J. G. J. & Bindels, R. J. M. Magnesium in man: implications for health and disease. Physiol. Rev. 95, 1–46 (2015).

2. Jiang, L. et al. Magnesium Levels in Drinking Water and Coronary Heart Disease Mortality Risk: A Meta-Analysis. Nutrients 8, (2016).

3. Michishita, R. & Ishikawa-Takata, K. Influence of Dietary Sodium and Potassium Intake on the Heart Rate Corrected-QT Interval in Elderly Subjects. J. Nutr. Sci. Vitaminol. (Tokyo) 61, 138–146 (2015).

4. Nicoll, R., Howard, J. M. & Henein, M. Y. A review of the effect of diet on cardiovascular calcification. Int. J. Mol. Sci. 16, 8861–8883 (2015).

5. Harrison's principles of internal medicine. (McGraw-Hill, 2012).

6. Haring, B. et al. Effect of dietary sodium and potassium intake on left ventricular diastolic function and mass in adults≤40 years (from the Strong Heart Study). Am. J. Cardiol. 115, 1244–1248 (2015).

7. Allen, A. R. et al. Dietary sodium influences the effect of mental stress on heart rate variability: a randomized trial in healthy adults. J. Hypertens. 32, 374–382 (2014).

7

MINERALS AND CANCER

Usually, human cells grow and divide to form new cells as the body needs them. When those cells grow old or become damaged, they die and new cells take their place. However, when cancer develops, old and damaged cells survive and new cells form when they are not needed. These extra cells divide without stopping and may form growths called tumors. Certain minerals may lower the risk for cancer or prevent a recurrence of cancer.[1]

MAGNESIUM (Mg)

There is some evidence that magnesium may reduce the overall risk of cancer. In one study, researchers found that the group with the highest magnesium intake seemed to have the lowest overall cancer risk, while the lowest magnesium level group carried a higher risk.[2] Another study examined different levels of magnesium intake in colon cancer patients compared to cancer-free patients. The lowest risk for colon cancer was observed with high-magnesium intake, while low-magnesium intake was associated with higher colon cancer risk. This equals a risk reduction of 24 percent for colon cancer and 18 percent for rectal cancer.[3]

Magnesium has also been shown to decrease the occurrence of reflux disease, a condition that can cause inflammation in the esophagus (potentially). Reflux and chronic inflammation are linked to an increased esophageal cancer risk.[4] Drinking water rich in magnesium has also been associated with decreased rates of esophageal cancers.[5]

Benefits of magnesium are notable whether they are from dietary food sources, magnesium-rich water or magnesium supplements.

The interesting thing about magnesium is that studies suggest it may have a protective effect against certain cancers, especially in the early stages. However, it should also be noted that certain cancer cells have a high affinity and requirement for magnesium, which may contribute to tumor progression in later stages.[6]

SELENIUM (Se)

Selenium may be protective against cancer, and a deficiency in this important mineral is a risk factor for several types of cancer. Research shows that low serum levels of selenium were found in lung, laryngeal, prostate and urinary cancer patients.[7, 8, 9]

CALCIUM (Ca)

Adequate calcium may decrease your risk for colorectal cancer. Recent studies confirm that high calcium intake is associated with a lower risk of colorectal cancer among both men and women. Maintaining the correct levels of calcium in your system could also reduce your risk for breast cancer as well.[10, 14]

ZINC (Zn)

People with increased dietary zinc intake may have a lower risk of lung cancer, a study suggested, noting the protective benefits of this mineral.[11]

COPPER (Cu)

People with increased dietary copper intake may have a lower risk of lung cancer, a study suggested, noting the protective benefits of this mineral.

IRON (Fe)

Increased iron intake may also help protect against lung cancer. However, excess iron intake can cause other health problems.[12]

SULFUR (Su)

Antioxidant enzymes glutathione peroxidase and glutathione reductase (which are sulfur compounds), catalase and superoxide dismutase (which is a manganese compound), all neutralize DNA-harming free radicals, which contribute to cancer development.[13]

REFERENCES

1. National Cancer Institute: What is cancer? https:/www.cancer. gov/about-cancer/understanding/what-is-cancer

2. Ko, H. J. et al. Dietary magnesium intake and risk of cancer: a meta-analysis of epidemiologic studies. Nutr. Cancer 66, 915–923 (2014).

3. Qu, X. et al. Nonlinear association between magnesium intake and the risk of colorectal cancer. Eur. J. Gastroenterol. Hepatol. 25, 309–318 (2013).

4. Song, J. H. et al. Oxidative stress from reflux esophagitis to esophageal cancer; the alleviation with antioxidants. Free Radic. Res. 1–20 (2016). doi:10.1080/10715762.2016.1181262

5. Liao, Y.-H., Chen, P.-S., Chiu, H.-F. & Yang, C.-Y. Magnesium in drinking water modifies the association between nitrate ingestion and risk of death from esophageal cancer. J. Toxicol. Environ. Health A 76, 192–200 (2013).

6. Castiglioni, S. & Maier, J. A. M. Magnesium and cancer: a dangerous liason. Magnes. Res. 24, S92-100 (2011).

7. Jaworska, K. A low selenium level is associated with lung and laryngeal cancers. PloS One 8, e59051 (2013).

8. Hurst, R. et al. Selenium and prostate cancer: systematic review and meta-analysis. Am. J. Clin. Nutr. 96, 111–122 (2012).

9. Borawska, M. H. et al. The effects of diet on selenium concentration in serum in patients with cancer. Nutr. Cancer 61, 629–633 (2009).

10. Abdelgawad, I. A., El-Mously, R. H., Saber, M. M., Mansour, O. A. & Shouman, S. A. Significance of serum levels of vitamin D and some related minerals in breast cancer patients. Int. J. Clin. Exp. Pathol. 8, 4074–4082 (2015).

11. Mahabir, S. et al. Dietary zinc, copper and selenium, and risk of lung cancer. Int. J. Cancer 120, 1108–1115 (2007).

12. Muka, T. & Kraja, B. Dietary mineral intake and lung cancer risk: the Rotterdam Study. Eur. J. Nutr. (2016). doi:10.1007/s00394-016-1210-4g

13. Amir Aslani, B. & Ghobadi, S. Studies on oxidants and antioxidants with a brief glance at their relevance to the immune system. Life Sci. 146, 163–173 (2016).

14. https://www.ncbi.nlm.nih.gov/pubmed/27466215. (Accessed: 31st October 2016).

8

MINERALS AND PAIN

Pain is a poorly understood human symptom of illness or injury. While some causes of pain are obvious, like a direct injury to a nerve, others, like migraines, are still mysterious.

What do we know about pain so far? Pain is part of a protective reflex. We have millions of neurons (the cells that make up the brain and nervous system) called nociceptors in our bodies. These cells receive signals about something being good or bad, then send signals to the brain. If it's something bad, your brain then thinks, "That was painful, I shouldn't do that," or, "I should call 911."[1]

When we pay attention to pain, like going to the doctor for chest pain, or ceasing running when the knee bothers us, it helps our overall survival. Because controlling pain is such a huge burden on the health care system, it's important to understand the science behind pain. Some of that science involves minerals!

MAGNESIUM (Mg)

Magnesium is one of the most interesting minerals with regard to pain and pain control. Animal and human studies show that magnesium has anti-nociceptor effects, meaning that it can keep the nociceptor from overreacting when it talks to your brain about the pain you are experiencing, whether it's a pulled muscle or a bee sting. For example, one study showed that rats who had surgery had less pain when they got morphine AND magnesium as opposed to just morphine. The rats' level of pain control was measured with the tail-flick test. The tail of the rat is heated until the rat flinches. The longer the rat waits before it flinches, the more effective the pain control.

In a human study of hip replacement patients, the humans actually experienced the same effect. Magnesium plus morphine was better than morphine alone.[2] Note that magnesium alone didn't reduce pain in rats or humans. So, you shouldn't take only magnesium after an operation or a major injury, but, adding a reasonable supplement, like 200 mg of magnesium citrate, could potentially help your pharmaceutical pain medication work better. As always, patients with heart or kidney problems or diarrhea should definitely discuss magnesium with a doctor first. Too much magnesium can worsen diarrhea, cause dangerous slowing of the heart, or overload failing kidneys.

You can also use magnesium as an effective remedy for muscular aches and pains. Many people use magnesium gels or lotions as a safe alternative to ibuprofen or acetaminophen. One study showed good benefits in leg cramps in pregnancy.[3] Magnesium is also a post-workout recovery ingredient for athletes who want to reduce muscle soreness time. Magnesium may help fibromyalgia as well.[4]

Many migraine sufferers take magnesium in order to prevent migraines. However, the Mayo Clinic issued a paper saying that supplements for migraines aren't totally proven. The clinic recommended that migraine sufferers focus on increasing the magnesium in their diets from nuts and vegetables. But migraine patients have been found to metabolize magnesium poorly and to have low levels of magnesium in the brain[5], and many patients would rather supplement to ensure that they get enough every day.

If you have migraines and your doctor agrees with trying magnesium, you can try supplements with increased magnesium-rich food consumption for a period of time to see how magnesium affects your symptoms.

POTASSIUM (K)

Like magnesium, potassium can also help with muscle cramps. When you sweat, you lose electrolytes, including sodium and potassium, and the loss of potassium can cause cramping. If you are going to be exercising hard for a long time, try to find a drink with some potassium in it or eat a banana before the workout. A study of male athletes found that the "post-race" banana was probably too late to help treat muscle cramps. The athlete's blood potassium levels didn't go up until an hour after eating one or two bananas, and even then, the rises were moderate.[6]

ZINC (Zn)

Zinc also has some promise in pain treatment. We know that it works powerfully on neurotransmitters—in the lab, zinc molecules influence the transmission of pain. Pharmacologists who wrote an article on zinc and pain are calling for zinc to be a supplement that goes with every prescription of Percocet, Vicodin, and Norco! Why? Animal studies suggest that zinc could help prevent opioid withdrawal and addiction, and we know that human patients "waste" the zinc in their bodies when they take opioids. The researchers saw these effects when they examined brain zinc levels in morphine-treated animals, and checked urine levels of zinc in opioid-taking humans.[7] Zinc has also been shown to help menstrual pain in teens.[8]

COPPER (Cu)

Copper may help with pain and anxiety, according to studies

on mice. While we don't have evidence yet that low copper means pain symptoms in humans, most multivitamins contain enough copper to take care of any deficiencies you may have.[9] But what about those copper bracelets for arthritis? Those have been studied, and unfortunately, it's a placebo effect.[10]

SODIUM (Na)

Researchers have recently established that some genetic mutations in sodium channels (the pathway by which the cells exchange sodium across the cell membranes) can cause pain syndromes. Some people with a mutation get somewhat lucky—they can't feel pain—while others have conditions that cause sudden bursts of severe pain, conditions that can run in a family. Of course, simply taking more sodium won't help these people—they need gene therapy or some way to fix or override the damaged cell structure. This is an area of research that interests scientists working on the problem of how to treat pain without opioids.[1] Similarly, potassium channel mutations can cause unusual pain syndromes. Expect to hear scientists talking more about these in the future.[11]

REFERENCES

1. Bennett, D. L. H. & Woods, C. G. Painful and painless channelopathies. Lancet Neurol. 13, 587–599 (2014).

2. Herroeder, S., Schönherr, M. E., Hert, S. G. D. & Hollmann, M. W. Magnesium—Essentials for Anesthesiologists. J. Am. Soc. Anesthesiol. 114, 971–993 (2011).

3. Supakatisant, C. & Phupong, V. Oral magnesium for relief in pregnancy-induced leg cramps: a randomized controlled trial. Matern. Child. Nutr. 11, 139–145 (2015).

4. Moulin, D. E. Systemic drug treatment for chronic musculoskeletal pain. Clin. J. Pain 17, S86-93 (2001).

5. Thomas, J. et al. Free and total magnesium in lymphocytes of migraine patients - effect of magnesium-rich mineral water intake. Clin. Chim. Acta Int. J. Clin. Chem. 295, 63–75 (2000).

6. Miller, K. C. Plasma potassium concentration and content changes after banana ingestion in exercised men. J. Athl. Train. 47, 648–654 (2012).

7. Ciubotariu, D., Ghiciuc, C. M. & Lupușoru, C. E. Zinc involvement in opioid addiction and analgesia – should zinc supplementation be recommended for opioid-treated persons? Subst. Abuse Treat. Prev. Policy 10, 29 (2015).

8. Zekavat, O. R., Karimi, M. Y., Amanat, A. & Alipour, F. A randomized controlled trial of oral zinc sulphate for primary dysmenorrhoea in adolescent females. Aust. N. Z. J. Obstet. Gynaecol. 55, 369–373 (2015).

9. Tamba, B. I., Leon, M.-M. & Petreus, T. Common trace elements alleviate pain in an experimental mouse model. J. Neurosci. Res. 91, 554–561 (2013).

10. Richmond, S. J., Gunadasa, S., Bland, M. & Macpherson, H. Copper bracelets and magnetic wrist straps for rheumatoid arthritis – analgesic and anti-inflammatory effects: a randomized double-blind placebo controlled crossover trial. PloS One 8, e71529 (2013).

11. 11. Mathie, A. & Veale, E. L. Two-pore domain potassium channels: potential therapeutic targets for the treatment of pain. Pflüg. Arch. Eur. J. Physiol. 467, 931–943 (2015).

9

MINERALS AND FATIGUE

Fatigue is something you may be familiar with. Numerous medical conditions such as heart, lung, liver and kidney diseases, hormonal disturbances, chronic lingering infections[1], mental and behavioral disorders, stress, nutritional deficiencies, immunologic problems[2], oxidative stress[3,4], sleep disorders and sleep apnea, inactivity, orthopedic conditions and pharmaceutical side effects may cause fatigue.[5] For a number of these conditions, fatigue could be an early and rather unspecific sign.

Some symptoms associated with fatigue include muscle pain or weakness, pain syndromes, which move throughout the body,[3,8,9] absence of a refreshing sleep[10], loss of memory and concentration[11], and unusual prolonged exhaustion for more than 24 hours after increased physical or mental activity. A newer study also suggests a connection between pain, fatigue, oxidative stress, and mitochondrial dysfunction while discussing medical reviews on fibromyalgia[3]. Minerals play an important role in combatting fatigue.

COPPER (Cu) AND ZINC (Zn)

Copper deficiency can cause decreased blood cell production, neurological impairments and fatigue.[12] Next to iron, copper is an essential mineral for red blood cells. Wilson's disease is an inherited disorder where increased amounts of copper get deposited to various tissues, such as the liver and brain, initially causing fatigue and nonspecific symptoms. As the disease progresses, it leads to liver cirrhosis.[22] Wilson's disease is treatable if diagnosed. Chelating agents can be used to bind to and excrete excess copper. Excess zinc can cause adverse symptoms in your body. Zinc and copper compete with absorption and carrier proteins. People who ingest unusually large doses of zinc can actually develop a copper deficiency, resulting in anemia and neurological problems.[19, 20]

Very high levels of copper are known to have toxic effects and can cause a variety of illnesses such as liver damage as well as central nervous system and kidney disorders. Initial symptoms may include fatigue, weakness, nausea, loss of appetite, vomiting and weight loss.[21]

MAGNESIUM (Mg)

Magnesium is needed by more than 300 human body enzymes to facilitate biochemical reactions. It helps create energy for the body, and activates muscle and nerve tissues by enabling potassium and calcium transfer through your cell membranes.[13] If magnesium levels in the body are too low, whole body systems don't work properly, resulting in fatigue and cramps in the early stages. It is estimated that a large number of people in the U.S. have low magnesium.

IRON (Fe)

Iron is an important element of your red blood cells. If the body lacks iron, your blood cells may not mature properly. The lack of iron may cause them to be smaller and unable to transport an adequate amount of oxygen to the tissues in your body. The resulting lack of oxygen may cause fatigue.

POTASSIUM (K)

Potassium is essential for cell function and normal blood levels are between 3.5 and 4.5 mEq/dl. There may not be any apparent symptoms when potassium is on the lower side or slightly deficient. However, further decrease in plasma and tissue potassium can have an adverse impact on a variety of cells, especially muscles and neurons. This can cause a myriad of symptoms, including fatigue. Decreased potassium intake, diarrhea, vomiting, chronic illnesses, water pills (diuretics), certain antibiotic side effects and excessive sweating all can lead to low potassium levels.[14]

CALCIUM (Ca)

Similar to magnesium, calcium impacts nerve conduction and muscle contractions. If calcium levels are inadequate, it can cause fatigue.[15, 16]

IODINE (I)

Iodine is an important building block of thyroid hormone. If the body does not have enough iodine, it cannot produce sufficient thyroid hormone. A poorly functioning thyroid is commonly linked with fatigue. [17, 18]

CAN EXCESS MINERALS CAUSE FATIGUE?

Zinc (Zn) and Copper (Cu)

Excess zinc can cause adverse symptoms in your body. Zinc and copper compete with absorption and carrier proteins. Persons who ingest unusually large doses of zinc can actually develop copper deficiency resulting in anemia and neurological problems.[19,20]

Very high levels of copper are known to have toxic effects and can cause a variety of illnesses such as liver damage, central nervous system and kidney disorders. Initial symptoms may include fatigue, weakness, nausea, loss of appetite, vomiting and weight loss.[21]

REFERENCES

1. Katz, B. Z. & Jason, L. A. Chronic fatigue syndrome following infections in adolescents. Curr. Opin. Pediatr. 25, 95–102 (2013).

2. Russell, L. Illness progression in chronic fatigue syndrome: a shifting immune baseline. BMC Immunol. 17, (2016).

3. Bazzichi, L. One year in review 2016: fibromyalgia. Clin. Exp. Rheumatol. 34, 145–149 (2016).

4. Galán, F., de Lavera, I., Cotán, D. & Sánchez-Alcázar, J. A. Mitochondrial Myopathy in Follow-up of a Patient With Chronic Fatigue Syndrome. J. Investig. Med. High Impact Case Rep. 3, 2324709615607908 (2015).

5. Fatigue: MedlinePlus Medical Encyclopedia. Available at: https:https://www.nlm.nih.gov/medlineplus/ency/article/003088. htm. (Accessed: 18th May 2016).

6. Loge, J. H., Ekeberg, O. & Kaasa, S. Fatigue in the general Norwegian population: normative data and associations. J. Psychosom. Res. 45, 53–65 (1998).

7. Lin, W.-Q. et al. Factors Associated with Fatigue among Men Aged 45 and Older: A Cross-Sectional Study. Int. J. Environ. Res. Public. Health 12, 10897–10909 (2015).

8. Goebel, A. Autoantibody pain. Autoimmun. Rev. 15, 552–557 (2016).

9. Klein, C. J., Lennon, V. A., Aston, P. A., McKeon, A. & Pittock, S. J. Chronic pain as a manifestation of potassium channel-complex autoimmunity. Neurology 79, 1136–1144 (2012).

10. McNicholas, W. T. Chronic obstructive pulmonary disease and obstructive sleep apnoea-the overlap syndrome. J. Thorac. Dis. 8, 236–242 (2016).

11. Cvejic, E., Birch, R. C. & Vollmer-Conna, U. Cognitive Dysfunction in Chronic Fatigue Syndrome: a Review of Recent Evidence. Curr. Rheumatol. Rep. 18, 24 (2016).

12. Miki, H. et al. [Copper deficiency with pancytopenia, bradycardia and neurologic symptoms]. Rinshō Ketsueki Jpn. J. Clin. Hematol. 48, 212–216 (2007).

13. NIH. Magnesium Fact Sheet. National Institute of Health Available at: https://ods.od.nih.gov/factsheets/Magnesium-HealthProfessional/.

14. Low potassium level: MedlinePlus Medical Encyclopedia. Available at: https://www.nlm.nih.gov/medlineplus/ency/article/000479.htm. (Accessed: 8th June 2016).

15. Cleveland Clinic. Hypocalcemia. Available at: http://www.clevelandclinicmeded.com/medicalpubs/diseasemanagement/endocrinology/hypocalcemia/. (Accessed: 8th June 2016).

16. Merck Manual. Hypocalcemia - Merck Manual. Merck Manuals Professional Edition Available at: http://www.merckmanuals.com/professional/endocrine-and-metabolic-disorders/electrolyte-disorders/hypocalcemia. (Accessed: 8th June 2016).

17. Iodine. Merck Manuals Professional Edition Available at: http://www.merckmanuals.com/professional/nutritional-disorders/mineral-deficiency-and-toxicity/iodine. (Accessed: 8th June 2016).

18. Symptoms and causes - Hypothyroidism - Mayo Clinic. Available at: http://www.mayoclinic.org/diseases-conditions/hypothyroidism/symptoms-causes/dxc-20155382. (Accessed: 8th June 2016).

19. Fosmire, G. J. Zinc toxicity. Am. J. Clin. Nutr. 51, 225–227 (1990).

20. Igic, P. G., Lee, E., Harper, W. & Roach, K. W. Toxic effects associated with consumption of zinc. Mayo Clin. Proc. 77, 713–716 (2002).

21. Wilson Disease. Available at: http://www.niddk.nih.gov/health-information/health-topics/digestive-diseases/wilson-disease/Pages/facts.aspx. (Accessed: 8th June 2016).

22. Lin, L., Wang, D., Ding, N. & Zheng, C. Hepatic Manifestations in Wilson's Disease: Report of 110 Cases. Hepatogastroenterology. 62, 657–660 (2015). 10 Vitamin and mineral deficiencies draining your energy http://dailyhealthpost.com/10-vitamin-or-mineral-deficiencies-related-to-fatigue/

10

MINERALS AND PREMENSTRUAL SYNDROME (PMS)

Bloating, ankle swelling, breast tenderness, pelvic pain, headache, fatigue, food cravings, moodiness, depression, poor concentration, crying and irritability. These are, of course, some of the most common symptoms of premenstrual syndrome, also known by its acronym, PMS. These symptoms are both physical and emotional, and often strike mid-cycle, ending when menstrual flow starts or shortly after. While they can certainly be frustrating and uncomfortable, they can also be quite severe. In fact, about 3-8 percent of these symptoms can be so debilitating that many women have missed a day or two of work. Severe PMS with depression, irritability and mood swings is called premenstrual dysphoric syndrome.[1-3] Medications are available to relieve some of the symptoms, but medications offer only temporary relief and have side-effects.

But what many women aren't aware of, and don't take advantage of, is that minerals can help reduce the severity of PMS symptoms.

CALCIUM (Ca)

The hormone estrogen controls the monthly cycle of women and also regulates calcium metabolism and absorption. Your hormones fluctuate during the menstrual cycle and so does your calcium.[2-4] These changes in calcium balance influence your mood, which may account for "PMS moodiness." It is therefore important that you be aware of your calcium levels and discuss your calcium intake with a competent doctor or nutritionist. Adequate calcium intake may also ease headaches, joint pains, fluid retention and some emotional disorders.[5,6] Calcium is the most well-studied mineral that may help PMS.

MAGNESIUM (Mg)

Magnesium is another mineral that has been shown to be effective in addressing PMS. Low magnesium may be a cause for PMS.[4, 7-9] A study of women who took 400 mg of magnesium a day saw vast improvements in their PMS symptoms. Ninety-five percent of them had less breast pain and weight gain and 89 percent had less nervous tension. Forty-three percent had fewer headaches too!

Fluctuating female hormones tend to make women more susceptible to magnesium deficiency than men. Hint: That's why many women crave chocolate before their period! Dark chocolate is rich in magnesium. Your body knows it needs more of this calming mineral.

POTASSIUM (K)

Potassium intake is highly associated with the occurrence of PMS, according to a big study of 1,057 women. This intake increased the risk of PMS in the study even at a lower intake than the current recommendaion of 4,700 mg/day. Potassium from the diet helps aldosterone, which is a hormone that fluctuates in menstruation and contributes to your PMS symptoms like bloating and water retention.[10] It may be wise to avoid extra potassium-rich food or supplements when you are menstruating.

CHROMIUM (Cr), COPPER (Cu), IRON (Fe), MANGANESE (Mn) AND ZINC (Zn)

Other minerals found to be imbalanced in women with PMS are chromium, copper, iron and manganese.[11] Low levels of zinc, iron, chromium and manganese were found in some studies of patients with PMS.[12] Copper was elevated and it competes with zinc in the gut; thus, your zinc intake should be higher to help with PMS symptoms.[9,13] Iron, especially from plants and supplements, was associated with a lower risk of PMS.[10] A study revealed that women with PMS may have a less nutritious diet, resulting in lower levels of the trace minerals (minerals you need in small amounts) that may help relieve PMS symptoms.

REFERENCES

1. Williams gynecology. (McGraw-Hill Medical, 2012).

2. Masoumi, S. Z., Ataollahi, M. & Oshvandi, K. Effect of Combined Use of Calcium and vitamin B6 on Premenstrual Syndrome Symptoms: a Randomized Clinical Trial. J. Caring Sci. 5, 67–73 (2016).

3. Tacani, P. M., Ribeiro, D. de O., Barros Guimarães, B. E., Machado, A. F. P. & Tacani, R. E. Characterization of symptoms and edema distribution in premenstrual syndrome. Int. J. Womens Health 7, 297–303 (2015).

4. Saeedian Kia, A., Amani, R. & Cheraghian, B. Erratum: The association between the risk of premenstrual syndrome and vitamin D, calcium, and magnesium status among university students: a case control study [Health Promotion Perspectives, 2015, 5(3), 225-230]. Health Promot. Perspect. 6, 54 (2016).

5. Ghanbari, Z., Haghollahi, F., Shariat, M., Foroshani, A. R. & Ashrafi, M. Effects of calcium supplement therapy in women with premenstrual syndrome. Taiwan. J. Obstet. Gynecol. 48, 124–129 (2009).

6. Thys-Jacobs, S. et al. Calcium supplementation in premenstrual syndrome: a randomized crossover trial. J. Gen. Intern. Med. 4, 183–189 (1989).

7. Whelan, A. M., Jurgens, T. M. & Naylor, H. Herbs, vitamins and minerals in the treatment of premenstrual syndrome: a systematic review. Can. J. Clin. Pharmacol. J. Can. Pharmacol. Clin. 16, e407-429 (2009).

8. Facchinetti, F. et al. Oral magnesium successfully relieves premenstrual mood changes. Obstet. Gynecol. 78, 177–181 (1991).

9. Posaci, C., Erten, O., Uren, A. & Acar, B. Plasma copper, zinc and magnesium levels in patients with premenstrual tension syndrome. Acta Obstet. Gynecol. Scand. 73, 452–455 (1994).

10. Chocano-Bedoya, P. O., Manson, J. E. & Hankinson, S. E. Intake of selected minerals and risk of premenstrual syndrome. Am. J. Epidemiol. 177, 1118–1127 (2013).

11. Torres, S. J., Nowson, C. A. & Worsley, A. Dietary electrolytes are related to mood. Br. J. Nutr. 100, 1038–1045 (2008).

12. Penland, J. G. & Johnson, P. E. Dietary calcium and manganese effects on menstrual cycle symptoms. Am. J. Obstet. Gynecol. 168, 1417–1423 (1993).

13. Quaranta, S., Buscaglia, M. A., Meroni, M. G., Colombo, E. & Cella, S. Pilot study of the efficacy and safety of a modified-release magnesium 250 mg tablet (Sincromag) for the treatment of premenstrual syndrome. Clin. Drug Investig. 27, 51–58 (2007).

11

MINERALS AND BEAUTY

Healthy levels of certain minerals may be a smart, long-term strategy for enhancing and preserving beauty.

SILICA (Si)

We have not discussed silica in its own chapter in this book. This is because we simply don't know what the recommended daily intake of silica is. This is what we do know: A deficiency of silica is associated with bone deformities, poorly formed joints, reduced cartilage, reduced collagen, and disruption of mineral balance in the femurs (thigh bones) and vertebrae. Collagen is like a protein meshwork that supports your skin like a bridge. Collagen is plentiful when we are young. Then as we age, the lack of collagen leads to sagging skin and wrinkles. Silica contributes to certain enzyme activities that are necessary for the formation of collagen. You can see how silica is important for young- looking skin.[1]

At least in animals, there doesn't appear to be a toxic upper limit to how much silica can be consumed. Multivitamins typically contain a little silica.

COPPER (Cu)

Remember how copper can be an antioxidant? Some researchers have created a chemical made from copper and chlorophyll—the green stuff in plants—and turned it into a topical skin agent for sun damage. According to their initial small study, the beauty treatment was able to reduce the aging caused by the sun damage to the skin.[2] (The product is called phytochromatic.)

SELENIUM (Se)

Selenium is also an antioxidant, and, as you might recall, can be very helpful or very toxic, depending on how much you take. One research group wanted to know if selenium was helpful or hurtful for skin sun damage. Human skin cells were blasted with UVA rays. As it turned out, the skin cells that were exposed to a certain form of selenium, selenomethionine, admirably resisted the damaging effects of the UVA rays—but only at low doses! This form of selenium actually made the UVA effects worse at very high doses.[3]

Selenium may have a role in preventing the inflammatory skin disease, psoriasis. A study that looked at the protein osteopontin, which is found in patients with psoriasis, found that high selenium levels were associated with low osteopontin levels and possibly better cardiovascular health.[4] Whether it's a coincidence or truly a clue to psoriasis is unclear, but keeping healthy levels of anti-inflammatory selenium is important.

ZINC (Zn)

Zinc has shown some promise as a treatment for acne. This skin condition can be quite persistent, at times retreating only to come back full force with a vengeance! In one study, taking zinc was associated with a 30 percent decrease in the number of acne lesions.[5] This is logical, because of zinc's anti-infective properties—acne is an infection of the skin. However, the amount of zinc used in the study was much higher than what we recommend, so to be safe, get your zinc levels tested. If you have persistent acne, stick to a safe amount of supplements, like 30 mg per day.

REFERENCES

1. Martin, K. R. The chemistry of silica and its potential health benefits. J. Nutr. Health Aging 11, 94–97 (2007).

2. Sigler, M. L. & Stephens, T. J. Assessment of the safety and efficacy of topical copper chlorophyllin in women with photodamaged facial skin. J. Drugs Dermatol. JDD 14, 401–404 (2015).

3. Hazane-Puch, F. et al. Six-day selenium supplementation led to either UVA-photoprotection or toxic effects in human fibroblasts depending on the chemical form and dose of Se. Metallomics 6, 1683 (2014).

4. Toossi, P. et al. Assessment of serum levels of osteopontin, selenium and prolactin in patients with psoriasis compared with healthy controls, and their association with psoriasis severity. Clin. Exp. Dermatol. 40, 741–746 (2015).

5. Göransson, K., Lidén, S. & Odsell, L. Oral zinc in acne vulgaris: a clinical and methodological study. Acta Derm. Venereol. 58, 443–448 (1978).

12

MINERALS AND MENOPAUSE

Menopause refers to that time in a woman's life when her ovaries cease to function optimally and she is not able to become pregnant. In the U.S., the average age for menopause is 51 years old.[1] Women are officially in menopause if they haven't had a menstrual period for one year.

While many women are happy to never buy a pad or tampon again, this transition may also cause unpleasant symptoms. Some women will experience hot flashes, night sweats, sleep difficulties, depression, mood swings and vaginal dryness. There is bone loss, weight gain, hair loss or thinning, forgetfulness, difficulty concentrating, skipped heart beats and muscle aches. Moderate to severe symptoms are often treated by hormone replacement therapies (HRT). However, with many hormone studies showing evidence of increased breast and ovarian cancer risk with HRT, as well as increased cardiovascular disease, many are weary about using them.[2] Antidepressants and anticonvulsants have also been used, but they can have side effects.

Menopausal symptoms can be debilitating and can affect quality of life. Minerals are being studied to help women through this stage of life when hormone replacement and other medications fall short or are not preferred as the first line of treatment.

CALCIUM (Ca)

Calcium is important in maintaining hair and nail health in perimenopausal and menopausal women.[2,3] Nail calcium has been found to be a good indicator of bone mineral density during menopause. In this age group, calcium loss in the urine is higher and absorption in the gut is lower emphasizing the need for a diet rich in calcium.[4]

The Women's Health Initiative (WHI) study found a higher hip bone density and lesser hip fractures in women taking 1,000 mg of calcium plus 400 IU of vitamin D a day.[2] The National Institutes of Health recommends calcium for the menopausal population to prevent osteoporosis, which is the thinning of bones that can start during this period.

However, some studies suggest that too much calcium may predispose women to cardiovascular diseases.[5] It can also increase hot flashes, especially in breast cancer survivors. In the WHI study, calcium with vitamin D did not improve hot flashes, mood swings or sleep problems.[6] Calcium has an established role in bone, nail and hair health in menopause, but you also need to consume healthy fruits and vegetables and increase your physical activity for overall health.[7]

ZINC (Zn), IRON (Fe), COPPER (Cu) AND MAGNESIUM (Mg)

Women who have low levels of zinc, iron, copper and magnesium may be at greater risk for menopausal osteoporosis.[8] Check your levels of these minerals and work with a qualified doctor to optimize them for your bone health.

SELENIUM (Se)

A drop in the levels of the hormone estrogen during menopause causes a drop in selenium levels.[9] This drop may contribute to an acceleration in aging, as selenium is an antioxidant. This decrease in selenium, however, is not seen in healthy menopausal women who consume a diet rich in selenium. It should be noted however, that increased selenium intake may have a negative effect on bone mineral density when calcium intake is less than 800 mg per day.[10] So, make sure you are getting all the minerals you need in a well-rounded diet.

Probably the most bothersome symptoms of menopause are hot flashes, mood swings and insomnia. Magnesium, zinc and iron may help with your mood swings, along with vitamin B6, according to many studies. Hot flashes, however, only showed improvement with hormone replacement. Calcium can make them worse.[2,6] (If you do not want hormone therapy but suffer from hot flashes, join a boot camp and exercise as regularly as you can. Exercising helps hot flashes, insomnia and your overall sense of wellbeing.)

Menopause is indeed a complex and inevitable change in all women. However, it can be a little simpler with a balanced diet and regular exercise to offset the mineral deficiencies that often arise during this important time, and alleviate many of its symptoms.

REFERENCES

1. Manson JE. Harrison's principles of internal medicine. - Menopause and Postmenopausal Hormone Therapy by Manson JE.

2. Chlebowski, R. T. et al. Calcium plus vitamin D supplementation and joint symptoms in postmenopausal women in the women's health initiative randomized trial. J. Acad. Nutr. Diet. 113, 1302–1310 (2013).

3. Goluch-Koniuszy, Z. S. Nutrition of women with hair loss problem during the period of menopause. Przegląd Menopauzalny Menopause Rev. 15, 56–61 (2016).

4. Ikeda, M., Ezaki, T. & Moriguchi, J. Levels of calcium, magnesium and zinc in urine among adult women in relation to age with special reference to menopause. J. Nutr. Health Aging 11, 394–401 (2007).

5. Li, K., Kaaks, R., Linseisen, J. & Rohrmann, S. Associations of dietary calcium intake and calcium supplementation with myocardial infarction and stroke risk and overall cardiovascular mortality in the Heidelberg cohort of the European Prospective Investigation into Cancer and Nutrition study (EPIC-Heidelberg). Heart Br. Card. Soc. 98, 920–925 (2012).

6. LeBlanc, E. S. & Hedlin, H. Calcium and vitamin D supplementation do not influence menopause-related symptoms: Results of the Women's Health Initiative Trial. Maturitas 81, 377–383 (2015).

7. Munshi, R., Kochhar, A. & Garg, V. Impact of Dietary Habits and Physical Activity on Bone Health among 40 to 60 Year Old Females at Risk of Osteoporosis in India. Ecol. Food Nutr. 54, 470–492 (2015).

8. Pedrera-Zamorano, J. D. et al. The protective effect of calcium on bone mass in postmenopausal women with high selenium intake. J. Nutr. Health Aging 16, 743–748 (2012).

9. Okyay, E. et al. Comparative evaluation of serum levels of main minerals and postmenopausal osteoporosis. Maturitas 76, 320–325 (2013).

10. Ohgitani, S., Fujita, T., Fujii, Y., Hayashi, C. & Nishio, H. [Nail calcium content in relation to age and bone mineral density]. Clin. Calcium 18, 959–966 (2008).

13

MINERALS AND DIGESTION

Our digestive system is a long tube stretching from the mouth to the anus. Organs like the liver and the pancreas hook into the tube to help us extract nutrition from food (like minerals) and eliminate contaminants (like toxic metals). Minerals play a part in keeping our digestive system healthy, helping it absorb the nutrients in our food, all of which are important for getting and staying healthy.

THE STOMACH AND INTESTINES

Sodium (Na)

Sodium is regulated by the kidneys, right? Not so fast! There's evidence that the gut may send the rest of the body signals about sodium before the kidneys encounter it. Case in point: When you take sodium orally, it's excreted more quickly than when it's given intravenously (IV). In other words, you would think that giving it IV, thereby bypassing the gut, is a quicker route to the kidneys, but the gut is the boss and tells the kidneys exactly how much sodium to save.[1]

Sodium can affect your fundamental gut balance as well. Chances are, you or someone you know has irritable bowel syndrome. This maddening disease features non-fun symptoms like bloating, cramping, and alternating constipation and diarrhea. As it turns out, sodium might play a role in IBS. There are cells in the intestines called the "cells of Cajal" that pump sodium across their membranes with a unique pump.

Genetic abnormalities in this pump are more commonly found in IBS patients – and may also cause heart problems! The gut might be "confused" by erratic electrical stimulation caused by the broken sodium pump. If you do undergo genetic testing and have IBS or heart problems, the mutation you are looking for is called SCN5A.[2] Remember that sodium is an "opposite" of potassium. Some scientists suggest that potassium transporters in the body could be where new IBS medications should act to encourage relaxation, not spasms and diarrhea.[3]

Potassium (K) and the Liver

There's a surprising connection with the liver and potassium as well. Liver injury or infection causes patients to urinate out, "waste," their potassium. When the liver heals, the potassium levels start to go back up.[4] This has implications for people with chronic liver problems, in terms of both their diet as well as their medications, since very low potassium levels can be more dangerous than the liver problem alone. If you have a liver infection or inflammation, ask your doctor what your potassium levels are, and whether you need a diet change or a pill to improve your status.

Zinc (Zn) and the Intestines

We're starting to see that when the body loses minerals in the food that you eat, problems arise! One of these problems is called acrodermatitis enteropathica, a genetic malabsorption of zinc through the intestinal cells. Losing zinc causes patients to get red and inflamed patchy areas of skin, inflammation of the nails, and hair loss. No wonder dermatologists recommend zinc for so many skin and hair conditions! Inflammatory diseases of the intestines like Crohn's disease can also cause zinc loss.[5] They cause the intestines to be so raw and inflamed that they can't effectively absorb nutrients.

Zinc can even treat a liver disease of copper excess called Wilson's disease. This fits what we've learned about zinc and copper balance. Children with Wilson's disease have been treated successfully with zinc.[6] Zinc is also recommended by UNICEF and the World Health Organization for treatment of diarrhea in children.[7]

Magnesium (Mg) and the Gut

Magnesium is also important in the gut. Good magnesium levels ensure proper motion of the gut, relaxing the muscles of the intestines so that food can pass through. That's why deficiency in magnesium often causes constipation. Oral magnesium, in a powder or pill, can help relieve this, although bath salts and topical oils and lotions can increase overall body magnesium levels as well. Calcium receptors, the attaching sites for calcium that trigger chemical reactions, are present in the part of the intestine closer to the head, while magnesium receptors are in the part closer to our feet.[8] Clearly, we have evolved to absorb calcium first! Based on how much calcium the body is "seeing," the body will then pull in the appropriate amount of magnesium from the gut to balance everything out. If you've consumed enough magnesium in the form of food and/or supplements, you should be calm, relaxed, and regular.

Magnesium may even prevent colon cancer, according to a meta-analysis done by a Chinese public health school after several studies seemed to hint at a link between higher magnesium intake and lower rates of colon cancer.[9] Another study indicated that 400 mg of magnesium per day is what is required for this protective effect (remember, that includes supplements and/or food).[10] This may be because of anti-inflammatory effects or just magnesium helping to move the bowels along every day. Magnesium also can help prevent colon cancer from toxic chemical exposure in drinking water, according to a Taiwanese study of colon cancer patients— an even better reason to protect yourself with supplements or increased dietary magnesium.[11] Meanwhile, high calcium levels are implicated in gastrointestinal cancers like esophageal, colon, and rectal cancer.[12]

Can magnesium be dangerous in the gut? Of course! Excessive oral supplements can lead to diarrhea, which can be dangerously dehydrating and lead to potassium losses. In one case, a patient ate magnesium citrate powder, but didn't drink any water. He ended up with chest pain and difficulty swallowing, and was found to have so much damage to the esophagus that he needed surgery![13]

If constipation isn't relieved by taking the recommended amount of magnesium, and the patient keeps taking magnesium, he or she can end up with hypermagnesemia, or high magnesium levels needing hospitalization. This condition can cause weakness and confusion and even heart problems and brain damage—just from taking too many supplements.[14] As always, there can be too much of any good thing.

Some medications can cause you to lose magnesium. Patients who use proton pump inhibitors (Prilosec, Prevacid, Dexilant, and more) for ulcers or heartburn should be aware that they are at risk of having lowered magnesium levels, since these drugs cause magnesium loss in the stool.[15]

THE PANCREAS

Your pancreas, a small organ located right behind the stomach, makes enzymes that process and digest food. The pancreas' tight regulation of minerals ensures that things in the GI tract work smoothly.

The pancreas makes an enzyme called caldecrin or chymotrypsin C, which deliberately lowers blood calcium levels by stopping the bones from leaching it out. Since leaching bones lead to osteoporosis, future patients may get infusions of caldecrin to treat osteoporosis.[16]

Many people think of diabetes as a "pancreas disease." While that refers mainly to type 1 diabetes, type 2 diabetes stems from dysfunction of cells in multiple structures and organs in the body. A full discussion of the interplay between minerals and type 2 diabetes is beyond the scope of this book, although magnesium does seem to increase the body's sensitivity to insulin[17], which is a benefit to type 2 diabetes patients. If you have type 2 diabetes, ensure that your magnesium levels are adequate.

REFERENCES

1. Lennane, R. J., Carey, R. M., Goodwin, T. J. & Peart, W. S. A comparison of natriuresis after oral and intravenous sodium loading in sodium-depleted man: evidence for a gastrointestinal or portal monitor of sodium intake. Clin. Sci. Mol. Med. 49, 437–440 (1975).

2. Verstraelen, T. E., Ter Bekke, R. M. A., Volders, P. G. A., Masclee, A. a. M. & Kruimel, J. W. The role of the SCN5A-encoded channelopathy in irritable bowel syndrome and other gastrointestinal disorders. Neurogastroenterol. Motil. Off. J. Eur. Gastrointest. Motil. Soc. 27, 906–913 (2015).

3. Currò, D. K+ channels as potential targets for the treatment of gastrointestinal motor disorders. Eur. J. Pharmacol. 733, 97–101 (2014).

4. Klevay, L. M. et al. Renal and gastrointestinal potassium excretion in humans: new insight based on new data and review and analysis of published studies. J. Am. Coll. Nutr. 26, 103–110 (2007).

5. Thrash, B., Patel, M., Shah, K. R., Boland, C. R. & Menter, A. Cutaneous manifestations of gastrointestinal disease: part II. J. Am. Acad. Dermatol. 68, 211.e1-33; quiz 244-246 (2013).

6. Abuduxikuer, K. & Wang, J.-S. Zinc mono-therapy in pre-symptomatic Chinese children with Wilson disease: a single center, retrospective study. PloS One 9, e86168 (2014).

7. Young, G. P. et al. Zinc deficiency in children with environmental enteropathy-development of new strategies: report from an expert workshop. Am. J. Clin. Nutr. 100, 1198–1207 (2014).

8. Lameris, A. L. et al. Segmental transport of Ca2+ and Mg2+ along the gastrointestinal tract. Am. J. Physiol. Gastrointest. Liver Physiol. 308, G206-216 (2015).

9. Chen, G.-C., Pang, Z. & Liu, Q.-F. Magnesium intake and risk of colorectal cancer: a meta-analysis of prospective studies. Eur. J. Clin. Nutr. 66, 1182–1186 (2012).

10. Gorczyca, A. M. et al. Association between magnesium intake and risk of colorectal cancer among postmenopausal women. Cancer Causes Control CCC 26, 1761–1769 (2015).

11. Kuo, H.-W., Peng, C.-Y., Feng, A., Wu, T.-N. & Yang, C.-Y. Magnesium in drinking water modifies the association between trihalomethanes and the risk of death from colon cancer. J. Toxicol. Environ. Health A 74, 392–403 (2011).

12. Wulaningsih, W. et al. Serum calcium and risk of gastrointestinal cancer in the Swedish AMORIS study. BMC Public Health 13, 663 (2013).

13. Assal, A., Saloojee, N. & Dhaliwal, H. Esophageal stricture due to magnesium citrate powder ingestion: a unique case. Can. J. Gastroenterol. Hepatol. 28, 585–586 (2014).

14. Weng, Y.-M., Chen, S.-Y., Chen, H.-C., Yu, J.-H. & Wang, S.-H. Hypermagnesemia in a constipated female. J. Emerg. Med. 44, e57-60 (2013).

15. Misra, P. S, Alam, A., Lipman, M. L. & Nessim, S. J. The relationship between proton pump inhibitor use and serum magnesium concentration among hemodialysis patients: a cross-sectional study. BMC Nephrol. 16, 136 (2015).

16. Tomomura, M. & Tomomura, A. Caldecrin: A pancreas-derived hypocalcemic factor, regulates osteoclast formation and function. World J. Biol. Chem. 6, 358–365 (2015).

17. Guerrero-Romero, F. & Rodríguez-Morán, M. Magnesium improves the beta-cell function to compensate variation of insulin sensitivity: double-blind, randomized clinical trial. Eur. J. Clin. Invest. 41, 405–410 (2011).

14

MINERALS AND ANXIETY

Anxiety disorders, defined as a subjective sense of unease, dread or foreboding, are quite common. Health care professionals report that they see anxiety in one form or another in about 20 percent of people looking for a medical provider. Anxiety may be part of a psychiatric illness or a reaction to a medical condition.[2] Recently, interest and research into the role of minerals in anxiety has been on the rise with initial promising results.[3-6]

ZINC (Zn)

Zinc is known to be one of the major minerals important in depression and anxiety.[7] Low zinc has been associated with oxidative stress, which is being studied as one of the causes of anxiety. Oxidative stress happens when there are not enough antioxidants to fight toxins and other harmful elements in your body. Zinc helps in fighting these free radicals or harmful elements because zinc has antioxidant properties.[1,4]

Multiple randomized controlled trials (RCTs) suggest that zinc may be an important mineral to consider when addressing mood disorders.[7] One of these trials studied a population with zinc insufficiency. It showed an improvement in depression and anxiety when blood zinc levels were increased.[1] Another study evaluated zinc and copper levels in 38 patients with anxiety and 16 without anxiety. Levels of the minerals, as well as antioxidants (vitamins A, E, C), were checked in the blood. The individuals suffering from anxiety had low zinc levels (and elevated copper) levels. [7,9,10] Zinc was given in oral form in those with depleted levels and anxiety symptoms improved significantly. Studies like these would suggest zinc plays a role in relieving anxiety symptoms and it may be important to work with your doctor to maintain an optimal zinc level if you have anxiety.

MAGNESIUM (Mg)

Because magnesium is needed in over 300 reactions in the body, its deficiency can have serious consequences, including triggering anxiety. [7–9] Studies have shown that magnesium deficiency may lead to depression and anxiety. A few trials have also shown that magnesium in combination with vitamin B6 may help lessen anxiety. High urinary magnesium was seen in a group of anxious subjects, indicating a lower magnesium blood level in these anxious patients. [10] Another large study of 6,000 participants revealed an increase in depression more than anxiety with a decrease in magnesium intake. [11] If you are feeling anxious, it might help if you eat a balanced diet, soak in an Epsom salt bath or apply magnesium gel or lotion to your body and get tested to see if you may need to increase your magnesium levels.

CALCIUM (Ca)

Few studies have been done on calcium and its effects on anxiety. High calcium can make your magnesium levels go down and this can make you more anxious. A study using a class of drugs that brought calcium levels down (calcium channel blockers) showed improvement in panic disorder. [12] These studies highlight the importance of regularly checking your mineral levels, including calcium.

MANGANESE (Mn) AND SELENIUM (Se)

Manganese can be toxic to the brain. [4,13] Studies disclose that chronic exposure to manganese may cause symptoms of depression, and high levels of the element have been seen in patients with generalized anxiety compared to controls. [13,14]

High levels of manganese accumulate in nerve cells, altering a substance called glutamate and this can cause excitation.

Low selenium is directly associated with an increased risk of depression, anxiety and other mental disorders.[6] A study done in a population with deficient levels of selenium in their diet showed improvement in mood and anxiety when supplemented with 100 mcg of selenium and the equivalent in their diet after five weeks.[15]

Lower selenium intake correlated with increased anxiety, depression and tiredness in the study. Supplementing with selenium may help lessen anxiety. The best way to determine whether supplementation is necessary is to consult your doctor and get tested.

REFERENCES

1. Russo, A. J. Decreased Zinc and increased copper in individuals with anxiety. Nutr. Metab. Insights 4, 1–5 (2011).

2. Kasper, D., Fauci, A. & Reus. Harrison's Principles of Internal Medicine, 19e. Mental Disorders, (McGraw-Hill, 2015).

3. Macpherson, H., Rowsell, R., Cox, K. H. M., Scholey, A. & Pipingas, A. Acute mood but not cognitive improvements following administration of a single multivitamin and mineral supplement in healthy women aged 50 and above: a randomized controlled trial. Age Dordr. Neth. 37, 9782 (2015).

4. Młyniec, K. et al. Essential elements in depression and anxiety. Part II. Pharmacol. Rep. PR 67, 187–194 (2015).

5. Lakhan, S. E. & Vieira, K. F. Nutritional therapies for mental disorders. Nutr. J. 7, 2 (2008).

6. Rao, T. S. S., Asha, M. R., Ramesh, B. N. & Rao, K. S. J. Understanding nutrition, depression and mental illnesses. Indian J. Psychiatry 50, 77–82 (2008).

7. Młyniec, K. et al. Essential elements in depression and anxiety. art I. Pharmacol. Rep. PR 66, 534–544 (2014).

8. Sartori, S. B., Whittle, N., Hetzenauer, A. & Singewald, N. Magnesium deficiency induces anxiety and HPA axis dysregulation: modulation by therapeutic drug treatment. Neuropharmacology 62, 304–312 (2012).

9. Lakhan, S. E. & Vieira, K. F. Nutritional and herbal supplements for anxiety and anxiety-related disorders: systematic review. Nutr. J. 9, 42 (2010).

10. Partyka, A. et al. Anxiolytic-like activity of Zinc in rodent tests. Pharmacol. Rep. PR 63, 1050–1055 (2011).

11. Jacka, F. N., Maes, M., Pasco, J. A., Williams, L. J. & Berk, M. Nutrient intakes and the common mental disorders in women. J. Affect. Disord. 141, 79–85 (2012).

12. Balon, R. & Ramesh, C. Calcium channel blockers for anxiety disorders? Ann. Clin. Psychiatry Off. J. Am. Acad. Clin. sychiatr. 8, 215–220 (1996).

13. Islam, M. R. et al. Comparative analysis of serum zinc, copper, manganese, iron, calcium, and magnesium level and complexity of interelement relations in generalized anxiety disorder patients. Biol. Trace Elem. Res. 154, 21–27 (2013).

14. Erikson, K. M. & Aschner, M. Manganese neurotoxicity and glutamate-GABA interaction. Neurochem. Int. 43, 475–480 (2003).

15. Benton, D. & Cook, R. The impact of selenium supplementation on mood. Biol. Psychiatry 29, 1092–1098 (1991).

PART II

MINERALS AS PART OF YOUR PROACTIVE HEALTH PLAN

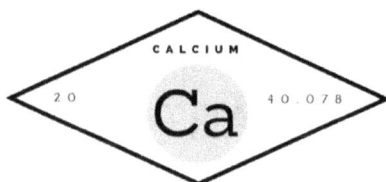

CALCIUM

Calcium is probably one of the most well-known minerals.[1,2] About 98 percent of your body's calcium is stored in your bones. You can find calcium in food, supplements and some medications, like antacids. The way your body absorbs calcium varies by age, with infants absorbing more than the elderly. Calcium is needed in many vital body processes like muscle contraction, bone metabolism, blood clotting, hormone release, neurotransmitters, and many more.

DIETARY SOURCES OF CALCIUM

Calcium can be found in many foods that compose our daily diet. Take a look at the following chart to see where you may be getting your calcium throughout the day – and how much you are getting.

SELECTED FOOD SOURCES OF CALCIUM

Food	Milligrams (mg) per serving	Percent DV*
Yogurt, plain, low-fat, 8 ounces	415	42
Mozzarella, part skim, 1.5 ounces	333	33
Sardines, canned in oil, with bones, 3 ounces	325	33
Yogurt, fruit, low-fat, 8 ounces	313–384	31–38
Cheddar cheese, 1.5 ounces	307	31
Milk, nonfat, 8 ounces**	299	30
Soy milk, calcium-fortified, 8 ounces	299	30
Milk, reduced-fat (2% milk fat), 8 ounces	293	29
Milk, buttermilk, low-fat, 8 ounces	284	28
Milk, whole (3.25% milk fat), 8 ounces	276	28
Orange juice, calcium-fortified, 6 ounces	261	26
Tofu, firm, made with calcium sulfate, ½ cup***	253	25
Salmon, pink, canned, solids with bone, 3 ounces	181	18
Cottage cheese, 1% milk fat, 1 cup	138	14
Tofu, soft, made with calcium sulfate, ½ cup***	138	14
Ready-to-eat cereal, calcium-fortified, 1 cup	100–1,000	10–100
Frozen yogurt, vanilla, soft serve, 1/2 cup	103	10
Turnip greens, fresh, boiled, 1/2 cup	99	10

Food	Milligrams (mg) per serving	Percent DV*
Kale, raw, chopped, 1 cup	100	10
Kale, fresh, cooked, 1 cup	94	9
Ice cream, vanilla, ½ cup	84	8
Chinese cabbage, bok choi, raw, shredded, 1cup	74	7
Bread, white, 1 slice	73	7
Pudding, chocolate, ready-to eat, refrigerated, 4 ounces	55	6
Tortilla, corn, ready-to-bake/fry, one 6" diameter	46	5
Tortilla, flour, ready-to-bake/fry, one 6" diameter	32	3
Sour cream, reduced-fat, cultured, 2 tablespoons	31	3
Bread, whole-wheat, 1 slice	30	3
Broccoli, raw, ½ cup	21	2
Cheese, cream, regular, 1 tablespoon	14	1

DV = Daily Value. DVs were developed by the U.S. Food and Drug Administration to help consumers compare the nutrient contents among products within the context of a total daily diet. The DV for calcium is 1,000 mg for adults and children aged 4 years and older. Foods providing 20 percent of more of the DV are considered to be high sources of a nutrient, but foods providing lower percentages of the DV also contribute to a healthful diet. The U.S. Department of Agriculture's (USDA's) Nutrient Database Web site lists the nutrient content of many foods and provides comprehensive list of foods containing calcium arranged by nutrient content and by food name.

** Calcium content varies slightly by fat content; the more fat, the less calcium the food contains.

*** Calcium content is for tofu processed with a calcium salt. Tofu processed with other salts does not provide significant amounts of calcium.[3]

RECOMMENDED DAILY INTAKE OF CALCIUM

Calcium needs vary by age. Newborns and growing children need 1,000 mg of calcium a day. This is obtained from breast milk, cow's milk and other dairy sources, like cheese. Adolescents need 1,000-1,300 mg a day, as they are still growing and are active.[4] Younger adults need about 1,000 mg. The requirements for calcium for older individuals are constantly changing. The recommended intake, according to the National Institutes of Health, is similar to that of adolescents.[2,5,6]

CALCIUM SUPPLEMENTATION

Calcium supplementation has been controversial. Some studies say that calcium supplements don't benefit bone health if your calcium intake is not poor to begin with.[7]

Calcium intake varies, but the average intake of most people ranges from 300-1,000 mg per day, according to a study, and this range did not cause problems. Supplementation may be needed if you are over 70 and are at risk for fractures, or have osteoporosis as seen in your Bone Density Test.[1,2,5,8] It is probable that if you are in this age group that you cannot absorb the calcium that you eat, or that you don't consume enough calcium. Recent studies suggest that calcium supplements may promote poor cardiovascular health. Thus, consuming calcium from food is best over supplements as long as your intake is enough.[6,8]

Vitamin D supplementation is needed in order for calcium to be utilized effectively by the body, especially if you are deficient. Testing is important to know your body's vitamin D levels.[9]

CALCIUM DEFICIENCY

Calcium deficiency happens when calcium is not moved from the bones to go into the blood and other cells. This is usually the result of kidney disease or parathyoid disorder (glands behind the thyroid, which help balance calcium in the body). This also happens in malnutrition as the gut also absorbs calcium. Another condition that may cause low calcium is a deficiency in vitamin D and an imbalance of the other minerals that bind to calcium, like phosphate, which need to be in the right proportion or else your calcium levels will drop. Calcium deficiency is often easy to treat and treatment depends on the cause.[5,10]

EXCESS CALCIUM

Having too much calcium in your blood is a condition doctors refer to as "hypercalcemia."[7] If your blood test results indicate that you have hypercalcemia, your doctor may recommend confirming it by repeating the test. You don't need to fast before testing your calcium levels. If it is confirmed that your calcium levels are elevated, your doctor should try to determine the cause in order to properly treat it.

Some causes of hypercalcemia include:

1. Primary hyperparathyoidism (an abnormally high concentration of parathyroid hormone, which regulates calcium levels in the blood, resulting in weakening of the bones through loss of calcium)

2. Lithium therapy (medicine for bipolar disorder)

3. Familial hypocalciuric hypercalcemia (related to decreased kidney release of calcium)

4. Vitamin D intoxication or too much vitamin D

5. High bone turnover like in hyperthyroidism, immobilization, vitamin A toxicity, and thiazides (used for high blood pressure)

6. Other conditions associated with renal failure like aluminum toxicity

Eating a calcium-rich diet is still the best way to meet your calcium requirements. Visit your health care provider and check your calcium levels.

REFERENCES

1. Institute of Medicine (US) Committee to Review Dietary Reference Intakes for Vitamin D and Calcium. Dietary Reference Intakes for Calcium and Vitamin D. (National Academies Press (US), 2011).

2. National Institutes of Health. Calcium - Dietary Supplement Fact Sheet.

3. United States Dept of Agriculture. Nutrient Data Laboratory : USDA ARS USDA. USDA National Nutrient Database for Standard Reference, Release 24 Available at: https://www. ars.usda.gov/northeast-area/beltsville-md/beltsville-human-nutrition-research-center/nutrient-data-laboratory/. (Accessed: 26th September 2016).

4. Mesías, M., Seiquer, I. & Navarro, M. P. Calcium nutrition in adolescence. Crit. Rev. Food Sci. Nutr. 51, 195–209 (2011).

5. Reid, I. R., Bristow, S. M. & Bolland, M. J. Calcium supplements: benefits and risks. J. Intern. Med. 278, 354–368 (2015).

6. Moore-Schiltz, L., Albert, J. M., Singer, M. E., Swain, J. & Nock, N. L. Dietary intake of calcium and magnesium and the metabolic syndrome in the National Health and Nutrition Examination (NHANES) 2001-2010 data. Br. J. Nutr. 114, 924–935 (2015).

7. Edgar V Lerma. Current Diagnosis & Treatment: Nephrology & Hypertension   Part 1 Fluid and electrolyte disorders. Chapter 6: Disorders of Calcium balance. (2009).

8. Meier, C. & Kränzlin, M. E. Calcium supplementation, osteoporosis and cardiovascular disease. Swiss Med. Wkly. 141, w13260 (2011).

9. Carmeliet, G., Dermauw, V. & Bouillon, R. Vitamin D signaling in calcium and bone homeostasis: a delicate balance. Best Pract. Res. Clin. Endocrinol. Metab. 29, 621–631 (2015).

10. Shin, C. S. & Kim, K. M. The risks and benefits of calcium supplementation. Endocrinol. Metab. Seoul Korea 30, 27–34 (2015).

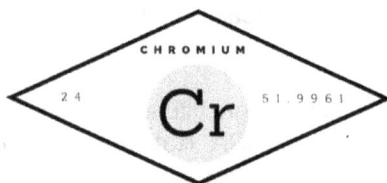

CHROMIUM

Chromium's benefits were discovered by mistake when a patient receiving liquid nutrition developed severe signs of diabetes, including weight loss and hyperglycemia (high sugar level), and increasing the doses of insulin didn't seem to help. Previous animal and preliminary human studies seemed promising, so the patient was given supplemental chromium. Within two weeks, the symptoms disappeared. This prompted researchers to look further into this mineral.[1]

Today, chromium is a popular mineral in sports supplements. In fact, people who exercise often tend to lose more chromium than those who don't. But this mineral is more than just a friend to athletes. It also may help keep type 2 diabetes at bay by reducing insulin resistance and maintaining healthy cholesterol levels. It even may prevent heart disease.[2-12]

DIETARY SOURCES OF CHROMIUM

You can find dietary sources of chromium in meats, whole-grain products, high-bran cereals, green beans, poultry, fish, broccoli, nuts, and egg yolk.[13]

RECOMMENDED DAILY INTAKE OF CHROMIUM

Age	Infants and children (mcg/day)	Males (mcg/day)	Females (mcg/day)	Pregnancy (mcg/day)	Lactation (mcg/day)
0 to 6 months	0.2				
7 to 12 months	5.5				
1 to 3 years	11				
4 to 8 years	15				
9 to 13 years		25	21		
14 to 18 years		35	24	29	44
19 to 50 years		35	25	30	45
>50 years		30	20		

https://ods.od.nih.gov/factsheets/Chromium-HealthProfessional/#h3

CHROMIUM DEFICIENCY

Life-threatening chromium defficiency isn't common. Human studies involving chromium deficiencies are difficult to establish since only small amounts are present in our bodies and the amounts may vary in different tissues.[15] Deficiencies may be estimated by lower levels of chromium in hair, nail, and plasma or urine analysis. The industrialization of our foods, with low levels of chromium in the soil, may be a contributing factor. The chromium in your diet may not be absorbed very well either – a problem that may only get worse with age. Additionally, foods high in simple sugars (sucrose or fructose) may cause you to excrete more chromium.

So, what happens when you have low chromium levels?

Well, one of chromium's key responsibilities is keeping your body sensitive to insulin, which means that chromium deficiency may increase your risk for diabetes. Low chromium levels are also associated with a higher incidence of metabolic syndrome and increased triglyceride levels.[3]

If you work out a lot, or you have issues with your blood sugar (including diabetes risk), you may want to get a lab test to check your chromium levels.[14]

CHROMIUM SUPPLEMENTATION

Chromium supplements are typically labeled to contain 200 mcg to 1,000 mcg per pill. Consumer Labs, an independent third party that tests supplements, found that some chromium supplements contain too little or too much chromium, and may occasionally contain harmful substances like lead, cadmium, arsenic and hexavalent (industrial) chromium. If you are found to be low in chromium, or if you are selecting a multivitamin that includes chromium, be sure to select a brand that invests in the research of their products before they put them on store shelves. Some of these supplement brands are only available through health care professionals.[15]

Overall, chromium supplements are well-tolerated by most people. It's been reported that some people experience cognitive or perceptual issues, headaches, insomnia, sleep disturbances, irritability, mood changes, low platelet or anemia syndromes, or liver and renal dysfunction. But it is unclear if these symptoms were related to the actual chromium or other potential contaminants in the supplement (another reason to choose the highest quality supplement possible!).

EXCESS CHROMIUM

No adverse effects have been associated with excess intake of chromium from food or supplements, but this does not mean that there is no potential for adverse effects resulting from high intakes. Because the data on the adverse effects of chromium intake are limited, exercise caution or talk to your health care professional before starting supplementation.

REFERENCES

1. http://care.diabetesjournals.org/content/27/11/2741.full. (Accessed: 31st October 2016).

2. Mertz, W. Chromium in human nutrition: a review. J. Nutr. 123, 626–633 (1993).

3. A scientific review: the role of chromium in insulin resistance Diabetes Educ. Suppl, 2–14 (2004). Bai, J. et al. Chromium exposure and incidence of metabolic syndrome among American young adults over a 23-year follow-up: the CARDIA Trace Element Study. Sci. Rep. 5, 15606 (2015).

4. Paiva, A. N. et al. Beneficial effects of oral chromium picolinate supplementation on glycemic control in patients with type 2 diabetes: A randomized clinical study. J. Trace Elem. Med. Biol. Organ Soc. Miner. Trace Elem. GMS 32, 66–72 (2015).

5. Yin, R. V. & Phung, O. J. Effect of chromium supplementation on glycated hemoglobin and fasting plasma glucose in patients with diabetes mellitus. Nutr. J. 14, (2015)

6. Balk, E. M., Tatsioni, A., Lichtenstein, A. H., Lau, J. & Pittas, A. G. Effect of chromium supplementation on glucose metabolism and lipids: a systematic review of randomized controlled trials. Diabetes Care 30, 2154–2163 (2007).

7. Wang, Z. Q. & Cefalu, W. T. Current concepts about chromium supplementation in type 2 diabetes and insulin resistance. Curr. Diab. Rep. 10, 145–151 (2010).

8. Bahijiri, S. M., Mira, S. A., Mufti, A. M. & Ajabnoor, M. A. The effects of inorganic chromium and brewer's yeast supplementation on glucose tolerance, serum lipids and drug dosage in individuals with type 2 diabetes. Saudi Med. J. 21, 831–837 (2000)

9. Dashkevich, O. V. et al. [Clinical assessment of dietary correction of metabolic syndrome by using specialized food product enriched with chrome]. Vopr. Pitan. 82, 30–36 (2013)

10. Suksomboon, N., Poolsup, N. & Yuwanakorn, A. Systematic review and meta-analysis of the efficacy and safety of chromium supplementation in diabetes. J. Clin. Pharm. Ther. 39, 292–306 (2014).

11. Ibarracin, C. et al. Combination of chromium and biotin improves coronary risk factors in hypercholesterolemic type 2 diabetes mellitus: a placebo-controlled, double-blind randomized clinical trial. J. Cardiometab. Syndr. 2, 91–97 (2007).

12. Huang, J., Frohlich, J. & Ignaszewski, A. P. The impact of dietary changes and dietary supplements on lipid profile. Can. J. Cardiol. 27, 488–505 (2011).

13. http://lpi.oregonstate.edu/mic/minerals/chromium. (Accessed: October 2016).

14. Bai, J. et al. Chromium exposure and incidence of metabolic syndrome among American young adults over a 23-year followup: the CARDIA Trace Element Study. Sci. Rep. 5, 15606 (2015).

15. Gibson, R.S. Principles of Nutritional Assessment. (Oxford University Press, 2005).

Additional Links:

• http://phlabs.com/chromium-a-promising-mineral-for-diabetes-treatment

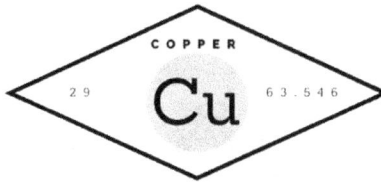

COPPER

$$\begin{array}{c} \text{COPPER} \\ 29 \quad \text{Cu} \quad 63.546 \end{array}$$

COPPER

We are so conditioned to think that consuming a metal is "bad" that copper doesn't sound like a nutrient at first blush. No wonder; lead, mercury, and antimony are poisonous! But, in appropriate amounts, our bodies definitely need copper.

Copper is a red-brown metal, a chemical element on the periodic table (Cu). Ninety-five percent of copper is carried around by a protein called ceruloplasmin. The rest is called free copper.[1]

In the body, it works by helping enzymes (proteins that trigger chemical reactions in the body) do their work. If there's enough copper around, these reactions will happen; if there isn't, fewer reactions will happen.

FUNCTION

One important type of reaction involves energy production in the body. Our bodies have little energy factories inside the cell, known as mitochondria, which create little energy packets known as ATP, from the food you eat. You need ATP for everything from getting up in the morning to digesting your food to thinking and pursuing a romantic partner! Without enough copper, mitochondria can't make enough of the ATP you need.

Copper functions as an antioxidant. Free copper is a positively charged entity that frequently "soaks up" electrons in the body. These loose electrons are also known as free radicals—and free radicals are famously damaging, causing aging and poor healing and immunity. But remember that this doesn't mean that more is always better. Too much of a good thing, and you max out the benefits of copper's antioxidant function and end up with toxicity problems.

Copper also is crucial for using iron in the body. For example, the copper enzymes called ferroxidases (not ceruloplasmin, which is pretty passive by comparison) carry iron to where it is used to make new red blood cells. In copper deficiency, iron literally gets stuck in the liver, which cause anemia. In the worst cases, the liver can be so overloaded with copper that the patient develops cirrhosis (scarring)!

Another important reaction is the linking of the proteins collagen and elastin. These proteins are the building blocks of healthy connective tissue, which does everything from making the skin appear plump to facilitating greater athletic ability (in the form of ligaments and tendons).

DIETARY SOURCES OF COPPER

Organ meats, shellfish, nuts, seeds, wheat-bran cereals, and whole-grain products are good sources of copper. One of our patients tested low on copper and remembered that she'd recently had cravings for oysters—which are high in copper and zinc! Sometimes your body can tell you what it needs.

RECOMMENDED DAILY INTAKE OF COPPER

The Linus Pauling Institute recommends an RDA of 900 µg/day for adults, and Pfizer (maker of the vitamin Centrum) calls 10 mg/day the safe upper limit. Centrum Women's contains 0.5 mg of copper, amounting to 500 micrograms. So, anyone taking this vitamin would still need food with copper in it!

COPPER DEFICIENCY

Copper deficiencies, as taught in medical school, arise more from genetic defects than from dietary reasons. But in reality, copper deficiency can occur in malabsorption, malnutrition, or very restricted diets like vegan or juicing diets without enough variety.

Surgeons have noticed that bariatric, or weight-loss/gastric bypass, surgery patients are more likely to have copper deficiency. The good news is it's usually not bad enough to cause symptoms. If you are planning to have bariatric surgery, consider increasing your dietary copper intake before the surgery and ask your doctor if you should get your copper levels checked after the surgery.[2]

Taking too much zinc (50 mg/day) can lead to copper deficiency, but taking a lot of copper doesn't seem to affect zinc. The reason is that zinc causes the intestines to make a protein that soaks up metals – and copper is a metal. Be sure not to soak up your copper, and read labels to ensure you aren't overdoing it on zinc. Many brands, like Nature's Bounty, sell 50 mg doses of zinc.

COPPER SUPPLEMENTATION

For people with low copper levels, taking a supplement may be a good idea. You can look for multivitamins that include copper, and add copper-rich foods to your diet with the help of a knowledgeable health care professional.

EXCESS COPPER

Excessive copper is usually caused by genetic defects, but some researchers suspect that copper in municipal water supplies could be increasing copper levels in people.

The classic disease of excess copper is Wilson's disease, which damages the liver and brain. Some suspect that it may be implicated in Parkinson's as well.[4]

Copper is likely involved in Alzheimer's disease, but researchers are still working out how. In a Turkish study, Alzheimer's disease patients had higher amounts of two metals – copper and manganese – in their hair than control patients. Hair analysis represents a longer period of time than a snapshot blood sample, so it may be more indicative that copper metabolism is abnormal in these patients. But does it mean that these patients "waste" more of their copper—i.e., it ends up in dead hair strands as opposed to being used in enzymes? Or is there some other explanation, such as people who eat more copper throughout their lifetimes end up with Alzheimer's disease? Meanwhile, selenium and zinc were lower in Alzheimer's patients' hair.[5]

In the lab, scientists have found that copper actually helps Alzheimer's "bad" brain protein—amyloid—stick to other clumps of amyloid. The whole thing sets off a toxic cascade that can accelerate the disease. As a result of this and other findings, some scientists think that increased copper levels are to blame for increasing rates of Alzheimer's.[6]

On a positive note, taking zinc supplements has been shown to lower copper levels in patients and slow down cognitive loss, and Alzheimer's patients tend to be zinc deficient. In this case, the copper-lowering effect is an advantage.[5,7]

TESTING

Copper or ceruloplasmin blood levels or urine levels are rarely tested for in the typical clinic setting. This is because most people get enough copper in their diets. However, your copper level can be tested along with "regular" blood work like cholesterol, and many specialty labs have micronutrient panels that test for copper. This can be especially important for signs and symptoms like unexplained anemia or weak, easily torn ligaments.

In general, scientists agree that testing for copper is unusually tricky. Age and other factors affect levels, and we do not have clear parameters for how much is unsafe or how much is optimal. We don't have proof that a certain level represents what the body is actually using in terms of copper. However, an abnormally high or low level, along with suspicious symptoms, might mean that trying a copper-containing vitamin (or cutting back on zinc and oysters) could be the next step in trying to treat the illness.

REFERENCES

1. Copper | Linus Pauling Institute | Oregon State University. Available at: http://lpi.oregonstate.edu/mic/minerals/copper. (Accessed: 3rd February 2016).

2. Nakagawa, M. et al. Assessment of Serum Copper State after Gastrectomy with Roux-en-Y Reconstruction for Gastric Cancer. Dig. Surg. 32, 301–305 (2015).

3. Venugopal, N. P. Approach to diagnosis and management of optic neuropathy due to copper deficiency. Neurol. India 63, 291 (2015).

4. Pal, A. Copper toxicity induced hepatocerebral and neurodegenerative diseases: an urgent need for prognostic biomarkers. Neurotoxicology 40, 97–101 (2014).

5. Koç, E. R. et al. A comparison of hair and serum trace elements in patients with Alzheimer disease and healthy participants. Turk. J. Med. Sci. 45, 1034–1039 (2015).

6. Hane, F. T., Hayes, R., Lee, B. Y. & Leonenko, Z. Effect of Copper and Zinc on the Single Molecule Self-Affinity of Alzheimer's Amyloid-β Peptides. PloS One 11, e0147488 (2016).

7. Brewer, G. J. Alzheimer's disease causation by copper toxicity and treatment with zinc. Front. Aging Neurosci. 6, 92 (2014).

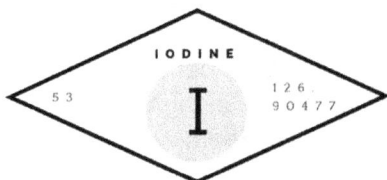

```
                    I O D I N E

         5 3         I        1 2 6
                              9 0 4 7 7
```

IODINE

The body needs iodine for some of its most fundamental functions. Iodine can make the difference between a healthy child and one with intellectual disabilities, or between a sluggish, obese person and a lean, vibrant one.

Iodine is important because it's used to make two hormones: T4 (storage thyroid hormone) and T3 (active thyroid hormone). These are both made in the thyroid gland, located in the neck. "Low" thyroid, or hypothyroidism, can cause problems including fatigue and a slowed metabolism. Some people can develop hypothyroidism from an iodine deficiency. No iodine, no thyroid hormones.

DIETARY SOURCES OF IODINE

Most people get their iodine from iodized salt. That's right—salt has to undergo a chemical process to turn into the Morton's free-flowing stuff. Beginning in the 1920s, iodine was added to the U.S. salt supply to prevent goiter—an enlargement of the thyroid gland that accompanies the low-iodine hypothyroidism. Salt was a logical choice, since everyone consumes it, it's not seasonal, and it's cheap to iodize it. Goiters improved as a result.[1]

Many countries require that table salt be iodized, but in the U.S., it's still voluntary for food companies to do it. But what if you don't use iodized table salt at home? Sea salt, with its greater taste punch, doesn't have any iodine in it. Not to worry.

There are many foods that contain iodine. If you consume dairy, you're getting iodine, all right – because the substance used to wash the cows' udders contains iodine! Strange, but it's an important 'accidental' source of iodine.[1]

Other than salt and dairy, there's iodine to be found in seaweed, like the nori used to wrap sushi rolls, and in seafood, potatoes, and navy beans.

RECOMMENDED DAILY INTAKE OF IODINE

The Institute of Medicine, a nonprofit organization providing guidance on science policy, recommends a daily iodine intake of 150 µg and a tolerable upper level of 1,100 µg in adults.[2] One sushi roll with seaweed contains 92 micrograms, so it's not too difficult to get your needed amount.

IODINE DEFICIENCY

As we've learned, thyroid hormone is essential to life and requires that enough iodine be around. Goiters and hypothyroidism can plague people who have low iodine levels, with symptoms including fatigue, constipation, hair loss, hoarse voice, puffy eyes, weight gain and disrupted menstrual cycles. Some people may be on prescription thyroid hormone pills for years, but not even realize that the culprit is low iodine, not a malfunctioning thyroid gland!

Pregnant women are particularly at risk for low iodine, since they tend to urinate their iodine (in iodide form) out more quickly than nonpregnant women. Without sufficient manufacturing of thyroid hormone, unborn children are at risk for cretinism, a severe form of developmental delay. Right now, pregnant women are not advised to take iodine unless they live in an area where everyone seems to have iodine deficiency (due to lack of access to supplemented salt, fish as food, or poor soil). However, this is controversial. Pregnant women, or people who are planning to become pregnant, can always request a urinary iodide level to make sure.[4] Based on the results, the doctor might prescribe a supplement or a diet change.

IODINE SUPPLEMENTATION

In general, it's rare that doctors recommend iodine supplements. It's easy to just purchase a container of iodized salt. It is virtually unknown for someone low in iodine to be getting too much sodium, so "too much salt" is typically not a concern. But for people who have difficulty converting inactive to active thyroid hormone, iodine supplements might be required. It's always best to check your levels and ask a doctor before taking iodine as a supplement.

Several studies have shown that kids who are iodine deficient start doing better in school and with cognitive tasks when they get extra iodine. In a Moroccan study, iodine-boosted milk improved schoolwork in elementary school children. Because some parents put their kids on very specific diets due to allergies or preferences, it's important to make sure that children are getting enough iodine by checking their levels or having iodized salt at home.[5]

IODINE EXCESS

Although it seems like having a lot of iodine around is good for the thyroid, the opposite can be true. Suddenly getting exposed to a lot of iodine, whether by binging on seaweed or getting a CT scan with (iodinated) contrast so the radiologist can see the body organs better, can throw the thyroid gland off for a while, causing hypo- or hyperthyroidism. Because of this, in Europe, some patients get a thyroid gland-blocking drug called methimazole before getting a CT scan with iodinated contrast. This practice is not usually done in the United States, however.[6] When patients with thyroid cancer are getting ready for treatment, they must consume a low-iodine diet to bring down their levels of thyroid hormone synthesis. The thyroid cancer cells are then "hungry" for iodine, and they greedily soak up the radioactive iodine, which kills off the cancer cells.[7]

REFERENCES

1. Pearce, E. N. National trends in iodine nutrition: is everyone getting enough? Thyroid 17, 823–827 (2007).

2. Institute of Medicine (US) Panel on Micronutrients. Dietary Reference Intakes for Vitamin A, Vitamin K, Arsenic, Boron, Chromium, Copper, Iodine, Iron, Manganese, Molybdenum, Nickel, Silicon, Vanadium, and Zinc. (National Academies Press (US), 2001).

3. Iodine in food and iodine requirements. Available at:http://www.foodstandards.gov.au/consumer/nutrition/iodinefood/Pages/default.aspx. (Accessed: 31st August 2016).

4. Andersen, S. L. & Laurberg, P. Iodine Supplementation in Pregnancy and the Dilemma of Ambiguous Recommendations. Eur Thyroid J 5, 35–43 (2016).

5. Zahrou, F. E. et al. Fortified Iodine Milk Improves Iodine Status and Cognitive Abilities in Schoolchildren Aged 7-9 Years Living in a Rural Mountainous Area of Morocco. J Nutr Metab 2016, 8468594 (2016).

6. Leung, A. M. & Braverman, L. E. Iodine-induced thyroid dysfunction. Curr Opin Endocrinol Diabetes Obes 19, 414–419 (2012).

7. Ju, D. L. et al. Dietary evaluation of a low-iodine diet in Korean thyroid cancer patients preparing for radioactive iodine therapy in an iodine-rich region. Nutr Res Pract 10, 167–174 (2016).

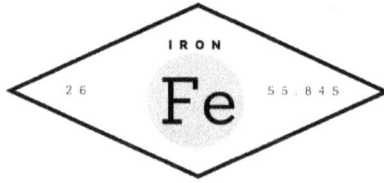

IRON
==

IRON

Iron is a critical mineral that every single cell in your body needs. It is needed to make hemoglobin, a component of your red blood cells that delivers oxygen to all the cells in your body. Without adequate iron, your body can't carry enough oxygen to your vital organs. Low iron levels may also leave you feeling quite tired.

Another reason why low iron = low energy? Iron-containing enzymes are responsible for energy production and metabolism.[1]

WHAT HAPPENS TO IRON IN THE BODY?

Iron absorbed from the gut is carried through the body in a protein called transferrin. About every hour, the iron carried by transferrin is delivered to the bone marrow to make hemoglobin. Though transferrin interacts with other cells in the body, like in the liver, the bone marrow has the most receptors. When iron levels are low, this iron delivery gets shortened to about 15 minutes to maintain iron in the blood, decreasing the bone marrow supply, and what follows is decreased production of oxygen-delivering hemoglobin, causing anemia.[1]

This iron deficiency can be caused by poor iron absorption in your digestion, blood loss like in menstruation, or red cell breakdown in certain diseases like malaria. After a certain time of having low iron, the red blood cell hemoglobin drops (anemia).[1]

An average adult male needs to absorb about 1 mg daily, and a woman in her reproductive years needs to absorb 1.4 mg daily. With iron deficiency, iron intake needs increase six- to eight-fold in order to continue healthy bone marrow production of hemoglobin.[1,2]

DIETARY SOURCES OF IRON

There are two types of iron – heme and non-heme. Heme iron is rich in lean meat and seafood. This is more bioavailable, meaning your body can use it better. Non-heme iron is found in nuts, grains, vegetables and other fortified products. The bioavailability (amount that gets absorbed) of iron from diets mixed with meat and seafood is about 14-18 percent, and about 5-12 percent in vegetarian diets. Absorption of iron happens in the gut and vitamin C enhances it. Thus eating vitamin C-rich foods when trying to build up your iron will help.

Men usually consume more iron than females, though females typically absorb more. Certain foods like grains and beans, which contain phytates (antioxidant compounds in grains, nuts and seeds) and phosphates, reduce iron absorption by half by binding to it.[3] When there is an excess iron from outside sources, a typical person's body can reduce its absorption, causing an accumulation of iron in your blood. This can cause iron toxicity, which can negatively affect important organs like the heart.[4]

IRON

SELECTED FOOD SOURCES OF IRON

Food	Milligrams per serving	Percent DV*
Breakfast cereals, fortified with 100% of the DV for iron, 1 serving	18	100
Oysters, eastern, cooked with moist heat, 3 ounces	8	44
White beans, canned, 1 cup	8	44
Chocolate, dark, 45%–69% cacao solids, 3 ounces	7	39
Beef liver, pan fried, 3 ounces	5	28
Lentils, boiled and drained, ½ cup	3	17
Spinach, boiled and drained, ½ cup	3	17
Tofu, firm, ½ cup	3	17
Kidney beans, canned, ½ cup	2	11
Sardines, Atlantic, canned in oil, drained solids with bone, 3 ounces	2	11
Chickpeas, boiled and drained, ½ cup	2	11
Tomatoes, canned, stewed, ½ cup	2	11
Beef, braised bottom round, trimmed to 1/8" fat, 3 ounces	2	11
Potato, baked, flesh and skin, 1 medium potato	2	11
Cashew nuts, oil roasted, 1 ounce (18 nuts)	2	11
Green peas, boiled, ½ cup	1	6
Chicken, roasted, meat and skin, 3 ounces	1	6
Rice, white, long grain, enriched, parboiled, rained, ½ cup	1	6
Bread, whole wheat, 1 slice	1	6
Bread, white, 1 slice	1	6
Raisins, seedless, ¼ cup	1	6
Spaghetti, whole wheat, cooked, 1 cup	1	6
Tuna, light, canned in water, 3 ounces	1	6
Turkey, roasted, breast meat and skin, 3 ounces	1	6
Nuts, pistachio, dry roasted, 1 ounce (49 nuts)	1	6
Broccoli, boiled and drained, ½ cup	1	6
Egg, hard boiled, 1 large	1	6
Rice, brown, long or medium grain, cooked, 1 cup	1	6
Cheese, cheddar, 1.5 ounces	0	0
Cantaloupe, diced, ½ cup	0	0
Mushrooms, white, sliced and stir-fried, ½ cup	0	0
Cheese, cottage, 2% milk fat, ½ cup	0	0
Milk, 1 cup	0	0

* DV = Daily Value. DVs were developed by the U.S. Food and Drug Administration (FDA) to help consumers compare the nutrient contents of products within the context of a total diet. The DV for iron is 18 mg for adults and children age 4 and older. Foods providing 20 percent or more of the DV are considered to be high sources of a nutrient.[4]

RECOMMENDED DAILY INTAKE OF IRON

For adults ages 19-50, women generally need 18 mg/day (27 mg during pregnancy and 9 mg when lactating), and men need 8 mg/day. The iron requirement for women ages 51 and up drops to 8 mg/day, just like men.[5]

IRON DEFICIENCY

Infants, children and adolescents may not be able to maintain normal iron levels in their bodies because of the demands of growing and their lesser iron intake. Breast milk has iron, but it is insufficient to meet a child's needs after four to six months.[6] The World Health Organization recommends supplementation in infants from 6-23 months of age when their diets are low in iron as children in this age group are often picky and poor eaters.

The American Academy of Pediatrics recommends supplementation only in infants who are primarily breastfed from four months old until they start eating iron-fortified foods. There is also a drop in iron in the last two trimesters of pregnancy.[9] Pregnant and nursing mothers should be proactive and ask their doctors about their iron levels and their child's iron intake.[7]

Cancer patients, those who donate blood frequently, women with heavy menstruation, those who have had gastrointestinal surgery like bypass surgery for obesity, and heart failure all may have depleted iron blood levels. In general, iron deficiency is not common in the United States except in certain lower-income areas where people don't get adequate iron from their diet, and in the above high-risk groups. If you have any of these risk factors, you should consider having your iron levels tested.

IRON-DEFICIENCY ANEMIA

Iron-deficiency anemia is the most common cause of anemia, especially in developing and underdeveloped countries. In the

U.S., this anemia is common in pregnancy, in blood loss, and in children because of poor diet. Symptoms depend on the severity of the deficiency, and they include pale appearance, fatigue, shortness of breath, small cracks in the mouth corners and spooning deformity of nails. It can cause cardiac arrest in the elderly with very low hemoglobin levels. It can also cause cognitive and immune system dysfunction. Diagnosis is by a simple blood test.[8]

When your iron levels become depleted, hemoglobin drops. Hemoglobin below 13 ug/dL in men and 12 ug/dL in women is considered anemia. Iron would also be measured, and normal is 50-150 ug/dL.

Treatment of iron-deficiency anemia includes correcting the cause of low iron and iron supplementation, either orally or through the veins. An iron-rich diet is also encouraged. Typically, supplementation is continued for 12 months. Oral iron therapy can cause digestive issues in some people, making their program difficult to stick with. Intravenous iron infusion may be done for you if you are unable to tolerate oral forms. More severe anemia would likely need a blood transfusion.

IRON SUPPLEMENTATION

Iron is available in multivitamins and multiminerals. Specific ones designed for women usually have 18 mg of elemental iron. Those that are geared toward men and seniors have less or no iron because of men's stores, and seniors' lesser need. Iron-only supplements provide about 65 mg, which is more than the recommended daily value. Forms of iron are often in ferrous or ferric salts. Ferrous forms are usually more bioavailable, meaning your body can use more of it.

Supplements with higher elemental iron, over 45 mg, can cause constipation and nausea. You will find different forms of iron in the pharmacy like carbonyl iron, iron amino acid chelates, and polysaccharide iron complexes. These have fewer gastrointestinal side effects and are more desirable.

Iron can interact with certain medications and minerals. Levodopa, which is used in Parkinson's disease, can be harder for your body to absorb when iron is taken with it. Levothyroxine, which is taken in thyroid conditions, can also be less effective with iron. Proton pump inhibitors like omeprazole, which decrease gastric acidity, decrease iron absorption. If you are taking any of these medications and you need to take iron supplements, please talk to your health care provider.[2,5]

Iron also decreases zinc absorption when the two are taken together. It is also recommended that calcium not be taken at the same time as iron, as it will also limit your iron absorption. Vitamin C, on the other hand, enhances its absorption. The important thing is to mention your use of iron supplements to your health care provider if you are also taking other medications or supplements.[1]

EXCESS IRON

Normal intakes of iron from food sources in healthy individuals usually won't cause any problems. However, iron intake from supplements of about 45 mg can cause gastric upset, constipation, nausea, abdominal pain and faintness, even if food is taken with it. There were cases of ingestion of 65 mg of iron that caused organ failure, coma, convulsions and even death. Iron supplements containing over 35 mg are required to have labels, stating an overdose can cause death. A few studies revealed that the elderly have higher stores of iron and are more likely to have a positive iron balance; thus, they don't need extra.[1]

If you are worried about your iron levels, contact a trusted health care professional and request a blood test. Iron supplementation is not for everyone.

REFERENCES

1. Harrison's principles of internal medicine, Iron Deficiency and Other Hypoproliferative Anemias. (McGraw Hill Education, 2015).

2. DRI: dietary reference intakes for vitamin A, vitamin K, arsenic, boron, chromium, copper, iodine, iron, manganese, molybdenum, nickel, silicon, vanadium, and zinc: a report of the Panel on Micronutrients ... and the Standing Committee on the Scientific Evaluation of Dietary Reference Intakes, Food and Nutrition Board, Institute of Medicine. (National Academy Press, 2001).

3. Gillooly, M. et al. The effects of organic acids, phytates and polyphenols on the absorption of iron from vegetables. Br. J. Nutr. 49, 331–342 (1983).

4. National Institute of Health. Iron - Dietary Supplement Fact Sheet.

5. Blanck, H. M., Cogswell, M. E., Gillespie, C. & Reyes, M. Iron supplement use and iron status among US adults: results from the third National Health and Nutrition Examination Survey. Am. J. Clin. Nutr. 82, 1024–1031 (2005).

6. Baker, R. D., Greer, F. R. & Committee on Nutrition American Academy of Pediatrics. Diagnosis and prevention of iron deficiency and iron-deficiency anemia in infants and young children (0-3 years of age). Pediatrics 126, 1040–1050 (2010).

7. Makrides, M., Crowther, C. A., Gibson, R. A., Gibson, R. S. & Skeaff, C. M. Efficacy and tolerability of low-dose iron supplements during pregnancy: a randomized controlled trial. Am. J. Clin. Nutr. 78, 145–153 (2003).

8. Recommendations to prevent and control iron deficiency in the United States. Centers for Disease Control and Prevention. MMWR Recomm. Rep. Morb. Mortal. Wkly. Rep. Recomm. Rep. Cent. Dis. Control 47, 1–29 (1998).

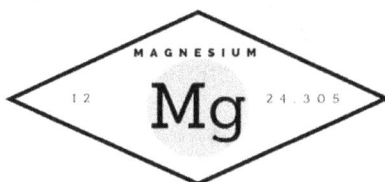

MAGNESIUM

Magnesium is one of the major minerals inside our bodies' cells. Outside the cells, it is an important cofactor for hundreds of processes and reactions in the body, including energy[1]. It is important in sugar breakdown and use, blood pressure regulation, and muscle and nerve function, including the heart muscle.[2–4] It contributes to bone metabolism (mature bone is removed and new bone is formed) and the synthesis of RNA and DNA, which are part of our genes. It also has antioxidant functions in more than one of the hundreds of reactions in the body that it is essential for. Anti-oxidation fights off toxins and other bad environmental hazards that can affect your body.

Most of your body's magnesium is stored in your bones. Outside the bones, most of it is inside cells. Of this, 95 percent is bound to proteins. The unbound form is the active form and is very little compared to what is bound. Measurement in the blood measures the unbound and is not an accurate measurement of total body magnesium. Magnesium is more accurately measured inside your cells, so tell your health provider that you want this test.

DIETARY SOURCES OF MAGNESIUM

Food sources of magnesium include leafy green vegetables (like spinach), legumes, nuts, seeds and whole grains. Foods with fiber are also good sources of magnesium. Many cereals are fortified with magnesium.

Some food processing, such as refining grains, actually lowers the magnesium content substantially. Tap, mineral and bottled water can also contain magnesium.[3]

RECOMMENDED DAILY INTAKE OF MAGNESIUM

Magnesium is abundant in many foods. Developed by the Food and Nutrition Board in the Institute of Medicine of the National Academies, the recommended daily allowance is the average amount sufficient to satisfy the nutrient requirements of nearly all healthy individuals.[4]

Age	Male	Female	Pregnancy	Lactation
Birth to 6 months	30 mg*	30 mg*		
7-12 months	75 mg*	75 mg*		
1-3 years	80 mg*	80 mg*		
4-8 years	130 mg	130 mg		
9-13 years	240 mg	240 mg		
14-18 years	410 mg	360 mg	400 mg	360 mg
19-30 years	400 mg	310 mg	350 mg	310 mg
31-50 years	420 mg	320 mg	360 mg	320 mg
51 + years	420 mg	320 mg		

MAGNESIUM DEFICIENCY

Causes of low magnesium include:[1,3,5]

1. Intestinal malabsorption conditions
2. Continuous vomiting and diarrhea
3. Defective kidney absorption
4. Poor magnesium intake secondary to alcoholism
5. Genetic disorders causing low magnesium and calcium
6. Poor absorption conditions

7. Certain medications like proton pump inhibitors such as omeprazole, and other medications affecting the kidneys like cisplatin, pentamidine, cyclosporine and aminoglycosides
8. Severe hypocalcemia (too little calcium) with low phosphate
9. Certain kidney diseases
10. Persistent loss of sugar in the urine in certain uncontrolled diabetics
11. Diabetic ketoacidosis (dangerously high sugar levels in diabetics that need hospitalization)[6]
12. Starvation
13. Rapid bone formation after parathyroidectomy, treatment of vitamin D deficiency, and bone metastases or cancer spread
14. Pancreatitis
15. Severe burns
16. Pregnancy and lactation
17. Severe sweating

Symptoms of low magnesium may include:

1. Neuromuscular symptoms like shaking, tremor, muscular weakness, imbalance when walking, spastic eye movements, vertigo, apathy, depression, irritability, psychosis and delirium.
2. Cardiac rhythm irregularities
3. Hypocalcemia (low calcium)
4. Hypokalemia (low potassium)
5. Headaches
6. Depression and anxiety[7]

Treatment consists of oral magnesium in the form of foods and supplements. More severe magnesium deficiency should be treated in the hospital with injectable magnesium. It is also important to give calcium, phosphate and potassium in some cases of low magnesium as these minerals balance each other in our bodies.

MAGNESIUM SUPPLEMENTATION[3]

Magnesium supplements come in different forms and absorption varies. The oxide, citrate and chloride forms may cause you to have loose stools. Thus these are often used in constipation while they also help in upping your levels. Magnesium oxide is the least absorbed form. Magnesium sulfate is the form in Epsom salt or magnesium bath salts. Aspartate, chloride, citrate and lactate forms are better absorbed than oxide and sulphate. The chloride form is in gels and lotions. The chelated (combined) forms glycinate and malate are the most readily available when you ingest them and thus are the best for low magnesium levels. High doses of zinc may interfere with absorption of magnesium supplements, so make sure you are not taking both at the same time.

Dietary surveys show that magnesium intake is lower than what is recommended in all ages in the United States. The elderly and adolescents are especially at risk of having lower intakes. For menopausal women, an error in supplementation is taking only calcium without magnesium. The ratio of intake should be 2:1 of calcium to magnesium. The federal government's 2015-2020 dietary guidelines suggest that nutritional requirements should be obtained mostly from food.

EXCESS MAGNESIUM

Causes of elevated magnesium include:[1,5]

1. Kidney disease as healthy kidneys can usually remove excess amounts of magnesium
2. Retention of large amounts of magnesium in intestinal diseases like in blockage or severe constipation and repeated laxative use
3. Severe trauma, severe burns, soft tissue injury, cardiac arrest, shock and blood infections that upset magnesium's balance

Symptoms may include:

1. Hypotension or very low blood pressure
2. Nausea
3. Lethargy
4. Lung failure
5. Coma
6. Paralysis
7. Gut sluggishness
8. Facial flushing
9. Pupillary dilatation
10. Cardiac rhythm abnormalities
11. Hypocalcemia (low calcium)

Treatment is directed at stopping the extra source of magnesium and correcting any problems that are hampering the natural removal of magnesium from the body.

Certain medications may interact with magnesium:[1,3]

1. Bisphosphonates (used in osteoporosis) – Magnesium can decrease its absorption. Thus you should take them two hours apart.
2. Antibiotics – Magnesium can interact with tetracyclines like demeclocycline and vibramycin, and quinolones like ciprofloxacin and levofoxacin. They should be taken two hours apart.
3. Proton pump inhibitors like omeprazole when taken for prolonged periods may cause magnesium levels to go down.
4. Diuretics or water pills like furosemide, bumetanide and hydrochlorthiazide may increase the removal of magnesium through the kidneys, causing magnesium depletion when used for prolonged periods.

You are probably convinced now of the importance of an optimal magnesium level in your body. It is very important for you to feel your best. If you are wondering if you should be taking magnesium, get tested and find out if you have sufficient levels, need to improve your diet, or need supplementation.

REFERENCES

1. Kasper, D. & Fauci, Antonio. Harrison's Principles of Internal Medicine, Chapter 423, Bone and Mineral Metabolism. (McGraw-Hill).

2. Mooren, F. C. Magnesium and disturbances in carbohydrate metabolism. Diabetes Obes. Metab. 17, 813–823 (2015).

3. National Institute of Health. Office of Dietary Supplements - Magnesium. National Institute of Health Available at: https:// ods.od.nih.gov/factsheets/Magnesium-HealthProfessional/. (Accessed: 28th September 2016).

4. Institute of Medicine (US) Standing Committee on the Scientific Evaluation of Dietary Reference Intakes. Dietary Reference Intakes for Calcium, Phosphorus, Magnesium, Vitamin D, and Fluoride. (National Academies Press (US), 1997).

5. Massy, Z. A. & Drüeke, T. B. Magnesium and cardiovascular complications of chronic kidney disease. Nat. Rev. Nephrol. 11, 432–442 (2015).

6. Barbagallo, M. & Dominguez, L. J. Magnesium and type 2 diabetes. World J. Diabetes 6, 1152–1157 (2015).

7. Tarleton, E. K. & Littenberg, B. Magnesium intake and depression in adults. J. Am. Board Fam. Med. JABFM 28, 249–256 (2015).

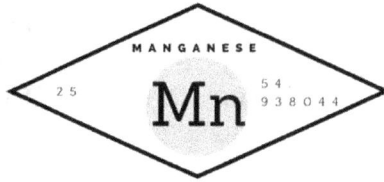

MANGANESE

It sounds similar to magnesium in name, but these metallic elements are totally different. Magnesium is needed in greater amounts in the body, for hundreds of functions and enzyme reactions. Manganese is a micronutrient that you only need in trace (small) amounts. Nevertheless manganese, named after the Greek word for magic, is a "must have" for good health.

Manganese is a hard, brittle, silvery metal, and it's the fifth most abundant metal in the Earth's crust. Including manganese in your diet is a must for antioxidant defense, energy metabolism and immune function. Manganese is involved in the formation of bones and in amino acid, lipid, and carbohydrate metabolism. It also helps to fight free radicals. Free radicals may occur naturally in the body but can damage cell membranes and DNA. They may play a role in aging, as well as the development of a number of health conditions, including heart disease and cancer. Manganese is also necessary for normal brain and nerve function.[1-3]

DIETARY SOURCES OF MANGANESE

Rich dietary sources of manganese include nuts and seeds, green leafy vegetables, tea, wheat germ and whole grains (including unrefined cereals, buckwheat, bulgur wheat and oats), legumes and pineapples.[3]

RECOMMENDED DAILY INTAKE OF MANGANESE

Based on the Food and Drug Administration's Total Diet Study for adult men and women, adequate manganese intake is 2.3 mg/day and 1.8 mg/day, respectively. The upper intake should cap out at 11 mg/day for adults. Overall, like other trace minerals, adequate intake of manganese is necessary, but high-dose intake is associated with toxicity.[3]

MANGANESE DEFICIENCY

Manganese is an important mineral for maintaining good health, especially because too little or too much of it can lead to some serious health issues. Here are some of the ways manganese deficiency can affect you.

Immunity

Manganese deficiency is associated with poor health outcomes. It causes depression of intestinal immunity, induction of inflammation and dysfunction of the intestinal physical barrier.[13,14]

Cancer Risk

There is an enzyme that is dependent upon manganese, called manganese superoxide dismutase. A recent study showed for the first time that a lack of this enzyme caused liver cell damage and an increased risk for liver cancer.[15,16,17]

Pregnancy

Pregnant women also need to be careful that they are not manganese deficient. Low (19 mcg/l) or high (26 mcg/l) manganese in your blood may coincide with a lower birthweight, compared to an optimum state of 22.5 mcg/l.[18]

Bones

Manganese is one of several trace elements necessary for bone health. It is believed that, among genetic factors, the female hormone estrogen determines up to 80 percent of peak bone mass in conjunction with environmental factors such as physical activity, medicine, smoking, being underweight, ovariotomy, alcohol drinking and nutrition. The process of bone formation requires an adequate and constant supply of nutrients, such as calcium, protein, magnesium, phosphorus, vitamin D, potassium and fluoride. There are several other vitamins and minerals needed for metabolic processes related to bones, including manganese, copper, boron, iron, zinc, vitamin A, vitamin K, vitamin C and the B vitamins. There is no specific evidence that manganese can prevent osteoporosis, but one study found that taking a combination of calcium, zinc, copper and manganese helped lessen spinal bone loss in a group of postmenopausal women. Lack of manganese causes impairment of cartilage growth and repair. [19-22]

Seizures

Several clinical studies suggest that people who have seizure disorders have lower levels of manganese in their blood. Nutrients that may reduce seizure frequency include manganese, vitamin B6, magnesium, vitamin E, taurine, dimethylglycine and omega-3 fatty acids.[35] Further studies need to be done to determine whether low manganese levels were the cause of the seizures.[34]

Diabetes

Mineral deficiencies may play a role in the development of diabetes mellitus, and that includes manganese. Blood and hair samples have shown that diabetics tend to have lower manganese levels, as well as zinc and chromium. It is unclear whether having diabetes causes levels to drop, or whether low levels of manganese contribute to developing diabetes. One clinical study found that people with diabetes who had higher blood levels of manganese were more protected from LDL or "bad" cholesterol than those with lower levels of manganese.[26]

MANGANESE SUPPLEMENTATION

Most people get manganese from their foods and will not need to take an additional manganese supplement. It is often included in supplements for bone and joint health, though. So, if you have bone or joint concerns, talk to your doctor about whether this option is safe for you to try.[20]

EXCESS MANGANESE

Although manganese is essential for normal cell function and metabolism, it can be toxic to the brain in high doses, especially on the developing brain. High manganese levels have been associated with lower IQ scores in children and increased rates of motor impairments.[27]

Manganese toxicity can cause muscle spasms and contractions. First described as "manganism" in miners during the 19th century, this movement disorder resembles Parkinson's disease characterized by hypokinesia (muscle rigidity and loss of muscle movement) and postural instability. [28-30]

Children exposed to higher levels of manganese as evidenced by blood levels, hair analysis and increased manganese water content showed impairment of certain neurological and cognitive functions, such as visual perception, memory and written language. Iron deficiency or a diet deficient in iron can lead to excess absorption of manganese, lead and cadmium, and can lead to neurodevelopmental impairments in children. [31]

Manganese toxicity is also associated with markers for oxidative damage and decreased kidney function.[31] Lastly, if you have excess manganese but you're deficient in magnesium, that's a double whammy. Magnesium deficiency can contribute to excess manganese and, therefore, increase the toxic effects of high manganese.

REFERENCES

1. Royal Society of Chemistry. Manganese - Element information, properties and uses | Periodic Table. Available at: http://www. rsc.org/periodic-table/element/25/manganese. (Accessed: 11th March 2016).

2. Tuschl K. Manganese and the brain. - PubMed - NCBI. Int Rev Neurobiol 110, 277–312 (2013).

3. Institute of Medicine (US) Panel on Micronutrients. Dietary Reference Intakes for Vitamin A, Vitamin K, Arsenic, Boron, Chromium, Copper, Iodine, Iron, Manganese, Molybdenum, Nickel, Silicon, Vanadium, and Zinc. (National Academies Press (US), 2001).

4. Dusek, P., Litwin, T. & Czlonkowska, A. Wilson disease and other neurodegenerations with metal accumulations. Neurol. Clin. 33, 175–204 (2015).

5. Fitsanakis, V. A., Zhang, N., Garcia, S. & Aschner, M. Manganese (Mn) and iron (Fe): interdependency of transport and regulation. Neurotox. Res. 18, 124–131 (2010).

6. Kim, Y. & Park, S. Iron deficiency increases blood concentrations of neurotoxic metals in children. Korean J. Pediatr. 57, 345–350 (2014).

7. Freeland-Graves, J. H. & Lin, P. H. Plasma uptake of manganese as affected by oral loads of manganese, calcium, milk, phosphorus, copper, and zinc. J. Am. Coll. Nutr. 10, 38–43 (1991).

8. Oregon State University. Manganese | Linus Pauling Institute | Oregon State University. Available at: http://lpi.oregonstate.edu/ mic/Minerals/manganese. (Accessed: 11th March 2016).

9. Manganese in Health and Disease. (Royal Society of Chemistry, 2014).

10. The effect of individual dietary components on manganese absorption in humans. - PubMed - NCBI. Available at: http:// www.ncbi.nlm.nih.gov/pubmed/1957822. (Accessed: 16th March 2016).

11. Freeland-Graves, J. H., Lee, J. J., Mousa, T. Y. & Elizondo, J. J. Patients at risk for trace element deficiencies: bariatric surgery. J. Trace Elem. Med. Biol. Organ Soc. Miner. Trace Elem. GMS 28, 495–503 (2014).

12. Friedman, B. J. et al. Manganese balance and clinical observations in young men fed a manganese-deficient diet. J. Nutr. 117, 133–143 (1987).

13. Schrutka L. Impaired High-Density Lipoprotein Anti-Oxidant Function Predicts Poor Outcome in Critically Ill Patients. - PubMed - NCBI. PloS One 11(3):e0151706, (2016).

14. Jiang, W.-D. et al. Manganese deficiency or excess caused the depression of intestinal immunity, induction of inflammation and dysfunction of the intestinal physical barrier, as regulated by NF-κB, TOR and Nrf2 signalling, in grass carp (Ctenopharyngodon idella). Fish Shellfish Immunol. 46, 406–416 (2015).

15. Konzack, A. Mitochondrial Dysfunction Due to Lack of Manganese Superoxide Dismutase Promotes Hepatocarcinogenesis. Antioxid. Redox Signal. 23, 1059–1075 (2015).

16. Xu, Y. et al. Manganese superoxide dismutase deficiency triggers mitochondrial uncoupling and the Warburg effect. Oncogene 34, 4229–4237 (2015).

17. Warburg, O. On the Origin of Cancer Cells. Science 123, 309–314 (1956).

18. Eum, J.-H. et al. Maternal blood manganese level and birth weight: a MOCEH birth cohort study. Environ. Health Glob. Access Sci. Source 13, 31 (2014).

19. Go, G. & Tserendejid, Z. The association of dietary quality and food group intake patterns with bone health status among Korean postmenopausal women: a study using the 2010 Korean National Health and Nutrition Examination Survey Data. Nutr. Res. Pract. 8, 662–669 (2014).

20. Palacios, C. The role of nutrients in bone health, from A to Z. Crit. Rev. Food Sci. Nutr. 46, 621–628 (2006).

21. Benevolenskaia, L. I. et al. [Vitrum osteomag in prevention of osteoporosis in postmenopausal women: results of the comparative open multicenter trial]. Ter. Arkhiv 76, 88–93 (2004).

22. Wang, J. et al. Effects of manganese deficiency on chondrocyte development in tibia growth plate of Arbor Acres chicks. J. Bone Miner. Metab. 33, 23–29 (2015).

23. Bolze, M. S., Reeves, R. D., Lindbeck, F. E., Kemp, S. F. & Elders, M. J. Influence of manganese on growth, somatomedin and glycosaminoglycan metabolism. J. Nutr. 115, 352–358 (1985).

24. Yen, J.-H. et al. Manganese Superoxide Dismutase Gene Polymorphisms in Psoriatic Arthritis. Dis. Markers 19, 263–265 (2004).

25. Hitchon, C. A. & El-Gabalawy, H. S. Oxidation in rheumatoid arthritis. Arthritis Res. Ther. 6, 265–278 (2004).

26. Kazi, T. G. et al. Copper, chromium, manganese, iron, nickel, and zinc levels in biological samples of diabetes mellitus patients. Biol. Trace Elem. Res. 122, 1–18 (2008).

27. Zoni S. Manganese exposure: cognitive, motor and behavioral effects on children: a review of recent findings. - PubMed - NCBI. Abstract Send to: Curr Opin Pediatr. 255–60 (2013).

28. Farina M. Metals, oxidative stress and neurodegeneration: a focus on iron, manganese and mercury. - PubMed - NCBI. Neurochem Int 575–94 (2013).

29. Remelli M. Manganism and Parkinson's disease: Mn(ii) and Zn(ii) interaction with a 30-amino acid fragment. - PubMed - NCBI. Dalton Trans 45(12), (2016).

30. Manganese Neurotoxicity: behavioral disorders associated with dysfunctions in the basal ganglia and neurochemical transmission. - PubMed - NCBI. J Neurochem (2015). doi:10.1111

31. Associations among environmental exposure to manganese, neuropsychological performance, oxidative damage and kidney biomarkers in children. - PubMed - NCBI. Env. Res 147:32–43 (2016).

32. Shin, D.-W. et al. Association of hair manganese level with symptoms in attention-deficit/hyperactivity disorder. Psychiatry Investig. 12, 66–72 (2015).

33. Hohle, T. H. & O'Brian, M. R. Magnesium-dependent processes are targets of bacterial manganese toxicity. Mol. Microbiol. 93, 736–747 (2014).

34. University of Maryland. Manganese. University of Maryland Medical Center Available at: http://umm.edu/health/medical/altmed/supplement/manganese. (Accessed: 16th March 2016).

35. Gaby, A. R. Natural approaches to epilepsy. Altern. Med. Rev. J. Clin. Ther. 12, 9–24 (2007).

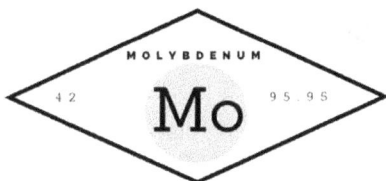

MOLYBDENUM

Here's a mineral you don't hear about too often: molybdenum. Molybdenum's actions are mainly in the production of enzymes, proteins that trigger chemical reactions in the body. These enzymes are involved in uric acid formation, transportation of iron, carbohydrate metabolism, and sulfite detoxification.[2]

Molybdenum is mainly found in the liver, kidneys, adrenal glands, bones, and skin, but exists in all body tissues. The body eliminates it in bile, urine, and stool.[1]

DIETARY INTAKE OF MOLYBDENUM

Some of the richest sources of molybdenum include lima beans, lentils, spinach, cauliflower, peas, and soybeans. You can also find it in whole grains, organ meats, wheat germ, oats, buckwheat, vegetables, and other beans. The body absorbs molybdenum well—up to 85 percent of the amount in green leafy vegetables gets absorbed into the body. Mineral-filled hard water can actually provide some molybdenum, as well.

RECOMMENDED DAILY INTAKE OF MOLYBDENUM

The recommended intakes of molybdenum are:[3]

- Adults 19 and older: 45 mcg/day
- Pregnant women: 50 mcg/day
- Lactating women: 50 mcg/day

MOLYBDENUM DEFICIENCY

Molybdenum concentrations are lacking in the soil of many geographic areas. In China, living in areas with poor molybdenum concentration has been linked to esophageal cancer, and the people living in these areas have low blood molybdenum.

Kids who are born with a genetic disease called molybdenum cofactor deficiency end up with a deficiency of three different enzymes. They can be born with developmental problems and aren't likely to survive to adulthood.[4]

In general, most people in areas without molybdenum deficiency in the soil don't have to worry. Molybdenum deficiency is uncommon, and you only need small amounts of this mineral, obtained through a healthy diet.

MOLYBDENUM SUPPLEMENTATION

Most multivitamins contain a small amount of molybdenum. The recommended daily allowance for adults is 45 micrograms, but most of us exceed that just from eating a regular diet. However, a review of popular diet plans, including the DASH diet, Atkins, and South Beach diet, found that these diets were low or completely lacking in molybdenum.[5] This underscores the importance of eating a balanced diet, not a fad diet.

MOLYBDENUM EXCESS

Animal studies have demonstrated reproductive and kidney problems with too much molybdenum; based on this, experts have decided that a good upper limit to consume daily for humans is no more than 2,000 mg. However, there have not been any clinical studies in humans confirming that this is the safe upper limit, though one individual who took high doses of a molybdenum-containing supplement developed hallucinations.[3]

Molybdenum does compete with copper in the body—there needs to be a balance between the two. Someone who takes a lot of one in supplement form runs the risk of a relative deficiency of the other.

One study found a link between poor semen quality and high levels of metals in the blood, including molybdenum. Molybdenum was high even when levels of the other metals were low.[6] More research in this area will be needed to determine if men should watch their molybdenum intake carefully when trying to have children.

REFERENCES

1. Lener, J. & Bíbr, B. Effects of molybdenum on the organism (a review). J Hyg Epidemiol Microbiol Immunol 28, 405–419 (1984).

2. Haas, E. M. & Levin, B. Staying healthy with nutrition: the complete guide to diet and nutritional medicine. (Celestial Arts, 2006)

3. Molybdenum | Linus Pauling Institute | Oregon State University. Available at: http://lpi.oregonstate.edu/mic/minerals/molybdenum. (Accessed: 5th April 2016).

4. Ichida, K., Amaya, Y., Okamoto, K. & Nishino, T. Mutations Associated with Functional Disorder of Xanthine Oxidoreductase and Hereditary Xanthinuria in Humans. International Journal of Molecular Sciences 13, 15475 (2012).

5. Calton, J. B. Prevalence of micronutrient deficiency in popular diet plans. J Int Soc Sports Nutr 7, 24 (2010).

6. Meeker, J. D. et al. Cadmium, Lead, and Other Metals in Relation to Semen Quality: Human Evidence for Molybdenum as a Male Reproductive Toxicant. Environmental Health Perspectives 116, 1473 (2008).

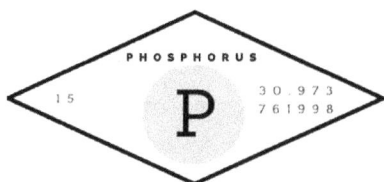

P

15   30.973
      761998

PHOSPHORUS

Though it doesn't have the celebrity status of calcium, phosphorus is almost as abundant in your body and is just as important. It works with calcium to build strong bones and teeth. It's also a key ingredient in the recipe for energy-producing ATP (adenosine triphosphate) in your cells, which means this mineral is important for how your body stores and uses energy. Phosphorus is also needed to make proteins like the one responsible for the oxygen-carrying capabilities of our red blood cells, and it is needed to repair cells.[1]

PHOSPHORUS

RECOMMENDED DAILY INTAKE OF PHOSPORUS

Table 1. Recommended Dietary Allowance (RDA) for Phosphorus

Life Stage	Age	Males (mg/day)	Females (mg/day)
Infants	0-6 months	100 (AI)	100 (AI)
Infants	7-12 months	275 (AI)	275 (AI)
Children	1-3 years	460	460
Children	4-8 years	500	500
Children	9-13 years	1,250	1,250
Adolescents	14-18 years	1,250	1,250
Adults	19 years and older	700	700
Pregnancy	18 years and younger	-	1,250
Pregnancy	19 years and older	-	700
Breast-feeding	18 years and younger	-	1,250
Breast-feeding	19 years and older	-	700

(Micronutrient Information Center of the Linus Pauling Institute)

DIETARY SOURCES OF PHOSPHORUS

Phosphorus is abundant in many food types. The main food sources are protein-rich foods like dairy, meat and fish. Most people get plenty of phosphorus in their diets.

Food	Serving	Phosphorous (mg)
Salmon (chinook, cooked)	3 ounces*	315
Yogurt (plain, nonfat)	8 ounces	306
Milk (skim)	8 ounces	247
Halibut (Atlantic or Pacific, cooked)	3 ounces	244
Turkey (light meat, cooked)	3 ounces	217
Chicken (light meat, cooked)	3 ounces	135-196
Beef (chuck eye steak, cooked)	3 ounces	179
Lentils** (cooked)	½ cup	178
Almonds**	1 ounce (23 nuts)	136
Cheese, mozzarella (part skim)	1 ounce	131
Peanuts**	1 ounce	108
Egg (hard-boiled)	1 large	86
Bread, whole-wheat	1 slice	68
Carbonated cola drink	12 ounces	41
Bread, enriched white	1 slice	25

(Micronutrient Information Center of the Linus Pauling Institute)
*A three-ounce serving of meat or fish is about the size of a deck of cards.
**Phosphorus from nuts, seeds, and grains is about 50 percent less bioavailable than phosphorus from other sources.

PHOSPHORUS DEFICIENCY

Deficiencies in phosphorus are primarily due to genetic disorders[1,3] These are diagnosed in infancy and often manifest with short stature in children afflicted. Bones are demineralized and softened due to the imbalance of phosphorus and calcium, which may cause bone conditions like osteomalacia and rickets.

Some of the other causes of low phosphorus levels (<1.0 mg/dL) include:[3]

1. Conditions causing alkalosis (conditions that make the body lose too much acid like vomiting or hyperventilation)
2. After carbohydrate ingestion and insulin injection
3. Large doses of aluminum and magnesium-containing antacids
4. Severe burns
5. Diabetic ketoacidosis (dangerously high glucose)
6. Inadequate phosphorus in hyperalimentation (feeding via a tube)
7. Alcohol withdrawal
8. Prolonged lung problems

Mild phosphorus deficiency rarely causes any major problems. Moderate to severe phosphorus deficiency can cause multi-organ failure. That's why it's important for you to be proactive and monitor your nutrient levels in your blood so you can address them before they become severe.

PHOSPHORUS SUPPLEMENTATION

Phosphorus in the blood is measured after fasting. If you are found to have low phosphorus, you may need to take an oral supplement with vitamin D. Intravenous supplementation (in your veins) is very risky as it can cause other problems like low calcium, low magnesium, low blood pressure and high phosphate. Thus, it is reserved for severely low levels of phosphorus and you will not get there unless you are very ill.

EXCESS PHOSPHORUS

High phosphorus levels can be due to:[4]

1. High phosphorus-rich food intake
2. Phosphorus laxative abuse
3. Intake of processed foods that use phosphorus additives
4. Decreased kidney elimination of phosphorus in renal disease
5. Cell death as in chemotherapy for leukemia or lymphoma

High intake of phosphorus-containing foods is especially bad if you have kidney disease. Restriction of protein-rich foods, however, is not recommended, according to many studies, as this causes malnutrition.[5] Thus, if your kidneys are sick, your health care provider will have recommendations for you to make sure your phosphorus levels remain within normal range.[6–8]

If your kidneys are well and you are healthy, high phosphorus by itself will not cause any damage to your body except for maybe its effect on your calcium level. Phosphorus may make your calcium levels go down when your phosphorus levels remain elevated for a long time. It may also alter the balance of certain hormones in your body. Your body will not work well when phosphorus is off. It is therefore important to keep your phosphorus levels balanced with the rest of your minerals and vitamins. When you visit your health care provider, make sure one of the tests you do is your phosphorus level.

REFERENCES

1. Butterworth, J. F., Mackey, D. C. & Wasnick, J. D. Morgan & Mikhail's clinical anesthesiology. (McGraw-Hill, 2013).

2. Calvo, M. S., Moshfegh, A. J. & Tucker, K. L. Assessing the health impact of phosphorus in the food supply: issues and considerations. Adv. Nutr. Bethesda Md 5, 104–113 (2014).

3. Carpenter, T. O. in Endotext (eds. De Groot, L. J. et al.) (MDText. com, Inc., 2000).

4. Nishi, T. et al. Excessive dietary phosphorus intake impairs endothelial function in young healthy men: a time- and dose-dependent study. J. Med. Investig. JMI 62, 167–172 (2015).

5. St-Jules, D. E., Woolf, K., Pompeii, M. L., Kalantar-Zadeh, K. & Sevick, M. A. Reexamining the Phosphorus-Protein Dilemma: Does Phosphorus Restriction Compromise Protein Status? J. Ren. Nutr. Off. J. Counc. Ren. Nutr. Natl. Kidney Found. 26, 136–140 (2016).

6. Beto, J. A., Schury, K. A. & Bansal, V. K. Strategies to promote adherence to nutritional advice in patients with chronic kidney disease: a narrative review and commentary. Int. J. Nephrol. Renov. Dis. 9, 21–33 (2016).

7. Kalantar-Zadeh, K. et al. Understanding sources of dietary phosphorus in the treatment of patients with chronic kidney disease. Clin. J. Am. Soc. Nephrol. CJASN 5, 519–530 (2010).

8. Murtaugh, M. A. et al. Dietary phosphorus intake and mortality in moderate chronic kidney disease: NHANES III. Nephrol. Dial. Transplant. Off. Publ. Eur. Dial. Transpl. Assoc. - Eur. Ren. Assoc. 27, 990–996 (2012).

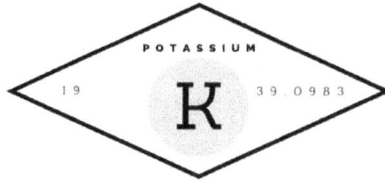

POTASSIUM

Potassium, often associated with bananas, is a must-have mineral. Potassium works with sodium to balance the fluids and electrolytes in your body, it helps keep blood pressure under control, and may help reduce kidney stones and bone loss as you age. It also may help decrease your risk for stroke. One recent study showed a link between white veggies and lower stroke risk, which is thought to be because of the veggies' high-potassium content.[1]

Potassium is also used to build proteins, break down and use carbohydrates to help fuel your body, build muscles, control the electrical activity of the heart and maintain the proper pH balance in the blood. In the brain, potassium helps nerve cells communicate with each other and with other parts of the body. In the muscles, potassium helps to tell the muscles when to contract.

DIETARY SOURCES OF POTASSIUM

High levels of potassium are found in figs, dried fruits (prunes and dates), nuts, avocados, bran cereals, lima beans, broccoli, peas, tomatoes, potatoes (especially their skins), sweet potatoes, winter squash, citrus fruits, cantaloupe, bananas and kiwi. Dried apricots contain more potassium than fresh apricots. Milk and yogurt are also excellent sources of potassium, as well as soy products and veggie burgers. Red meat, chicken and fish such as salmon, cod, flounder and sardines are also good sources of potassium. While potatoes are the highest source of dietary potassium, the addition of salt should be limited.[4-6]

RECOMMENDED DAILY INTAKE OF POTASSIUM

Generally, you should aim for 4.7g (120 mmol) of potassium per day. Unfortunately, potassium is one of those nutrients that many people don't get enough of. In fact, many people only get half the recommended daily value. This may be part of the problem in the U.S. with high blood pressure, which is sometimes associated with low potassium levels.

Western diets traditionally include limited potassium intake with reduced consumption of fruits and vegetables, paired with an increase in sodium intake through increased consumption of processed foods. In recent surveys, the median intake of potassium by adults in the United States was approximately 2.8 to 3.3 g per day for men and 2.2 to 2.4 g per day for women; in Canada, the median intakes ranged from 3.2 to 3.4 g per day for men and 2.4 to 2.6 g per day for women.[2-3]

POTASSIUM DEFICIENCY

Low potassium levels may go unrecognized and without symptoms. More pronounced loss of potassium can cause muscle and general weakness, tingling, numbness, twitches, paralysis, palpitations and abnormal heart rhythm, fainting, depression, confusion, delirium, hallucinations, abdominal cramping or constipation.

In healthy people, approximately 85 percent of dietary potassium is absorbed. Magnesium is an important co-factor in absorption. If magnesium levels are low, it affects potassium as well, causing decreased absorption and lower levels. Causes for low potassium may include diarrhea or vomiting, kidney disorders, frequent laxative or enema use, or medication side effects (diuretics, steroids, aminoglycoside antibiotics). People who don't get a lot of potassium in their diets may be at risk for deficiency.

A high-sodium, low-potassium diet is associated with a 50 percent increase in all-cause mortality (i.e., death). High potassium intake by itself was shown to have 20 percent lower mortality rate.

One reason potassium deficiency is so harmful? Potassium deficiency may increase your blood pressure. Low potassium also increases salt sensitivity. A 2012 study reported that one third of Americans have high blood pressure, accounting for one of every 6 deaths in 2005. This is no small issue!

Many scientific studies have suggested that an increase in potassium may lower high blood pressure, also called hypertension. The magnitude of the blood pressure-lowering effect is greater in patients with high blood pressure, and appears to be more pronounced the longer the duration of the supplementation.

Diets rich in vegetables, fruits and low-fat dairy products may improve blood pressure by 11.4 mm systolic and 5.5 mm diastolic, research shows, compared to diets low in vegetables, low in fruits and with regular dairy.

Besides high blood pressure, another symptom of potassium deficiency is getting those pesky leg cramps. Marathon runners have been known to experience leg cramps as their muscles are pushed to the limits and they sweat out their precious electrolytes, including potassium. Based on an average loss of 4-8 mmol/L sweat, this converts to a loss of 100-200 mg (or 1-2 g) of potassium per hour for an average adult during activity. This is why they are often handed a banana! In fact, too little potassium, calcium or magnesium can contribute to leg cramps (not only potassium), so if you are exercising, make sure you have a sports drink that addresses all of these needs. Medications prescribed for hypertension called diuretics can also deplete your potassium.[13-16]

POTASSIUM SUPPLEMENTATION

For people with low potassium, taking a potassium supplement may be a good idea. Based on the results of a lab test, depending how deficient in potassium you are, a knowledgeable health care professional can recommend the appropriate dose to bring your levels back to normal.

Adding a potassium supplement to your diet may offset some of the harmful effects of a sodium-rich meal. In addition, supplementing with potassium bicarbonate can improve bone metabolism and keep a bone healthy longer. This is partially achieved by creating a more alkaline environment, counteracting the loss of bone minerals. Alkaline diets with low acidity, such as vegan diets, can also achieve the same effect.[19]

EXCESS POTASSIUM

The kidneys play an important role in retaining potassium when levels are low or excreting it when levels are high. If your kidneys are not working properly, you can accumulate excess potassium – typical for dialysis patients.

Excess potassium may have no symptoms in the initial phases; however, it can lead to nausea, heart rhythm irregularities and, in very high doses, heart block. Causes of excess potassium are most common among patients with kidney failure and their impaired ability to excrete potassium, excess IV infusion or excess oral intake. It can be caused by intracellular (inside the cells) release of potassium from damaged cells, caused by traumatic injuries, large burns, drugs, surgery, certain anemias and infection.

Small elevations in your potassium levels are mostly inconsequential and can be addressed by avoiding potassium-rich foods until levels come back to normal, or in some cases, you may need potassium-binding agents, such as kayexailate, to decrease absorption. It may require stopping any drugs that cause increased potassium as side effect, such as certain diuretics and blood pressure pills. Inability to excrete potassium through the kidneys may require dialysis.

REFERENCES

1. Medline Plus. Potassium - Element information, properties and uses | Periodic Table. Royal Society of Chemistry Available at: http://www.rsc.org/periodic-table/element/19/potassium. (Accessed: 26th February 2016).

2. Institute of Medicine of the National Academies, P. on D. R. I. for E. and W. Dietary Reference Intakes for Water, Potassium, Sodium, Chloride, and Sulfate. (National Academies Press, 2005).

3. Weaver, C. M. Potassium and Health123. Adv. Nutr. 4, 368S–377S (2013).

4. National Institue of Health. Potassium in diet: MedlinePlus Medical Encyclopedia. Available at: https://www.nlm.nih.gov/medlineplus/ency/article/002413.htm. (Accessed: 24th February 2016).

5. Cohn JN, Kowey PR, Whelton PK & Prisant L. New guidelines for potassium replacement in clinical practice: A contemporary review by the national council on potassium in clinical practice. Arch. Intern. Med. 160, 2429–2436 (2000).

6. Tizioto, P. C. et al. Calcium and potassium content in beef: influences on tenderness and associations with molecular markers in Nellore cattle. Meat Sci. 96, 436–440 (2014).

7. An Integrated View of Potassium Homeostasis — NEJM. New England Journal of Medicine Available at: http://www.nejm.org/doi/full/10.1056/NEJMc1509656. (Accessed: 16th January 2016).

8. Sebastian, A., Harris, S. T., Ottaway, J. H., Todd, K. M. & Morris, R. C. Improved mineral balance and skeletal metabolism in postmenopausal women treated with potassium bicarbonate. N. Engl. J. Med. 330, 1776–1781 (1994).

9. Sebastian, A. & Frassetto, L. A. Estimation of the net acid load of the diet of ancestral preagricultural Homo sapiens and their hominid ancestors. Am. J. Clin. Nutr. 76, 1308–1316 (2002).

10. Sebastian, A., Frassetto, L. A., Sellmeyer, D. E. & Morris, R. C. The evolution-informed optimal dietary potassium intake of human beings greatly exceeds current and recommended intakes. Semin. Nephrol. 26, 447–453 (2006).

11. Yang, Q. & Liu, T. Sodium and potassium intake and mortality among US adults: prospective data from the Third National Health and Nutrition Examination Survey. Arch. Intern. Med. 171, 1183–1191 (2011).

12. Cook, N. R. et al. Joint effects of sodium and potassium intake on subsequent cardiovascular disease: the Trials of Hypertension Prevention follow-up study. Arch. Intern. Med. 169, 32–40 (2009).

13. Whelton, P. K. et al. Effects of oral potassium on blood pressure. Meta-analysis of randomized controlled clinical trials. JAMA 277, 1624–1632 (1997).

14. Cappuccio, F. P. & MacGregor, G. A. Does potassium supplementation lower blood pressure? A meta-analysis of published trials. J. Hypertens. 9, 465–473 (1991).

15. Roger, V. L. et al. Heart disease and stroke statistics – 2012 update: a report from the American Heart Association. Circulation 125, e2–e220 (2012).

16. Appel, L. J. & Moore, T. J. A clinical trial of the effects of dietary patterns on blood pressure. DASH Collaborative Research Group. N. Engl. J. Med. 336, 1117–1124 (1997).

17. Blanch, N., Clifton, P. M., Petersen, K. S. & Keogh, J. B. Effect of sodium and potassium supplementation on vascular and endothelial function: a randomized controlled trial. Am. J. Clin. Nutr. 101, 939–946 (2015).

18. Blanch, N., Clifton, P. M. & Keogh, J. B. Postprandial effects of potassium supplementation on vascular function and blood pressure: a randomized cross-over study. Nutr. Metab. Cardiovasc. Dis. NMCD 24, 148–154 (2014).

19. Burckhardt, P. The role of low acid load in vegetarian diet on bone health: a narrative review. Swiss Med. Wkly. 146, w14277 (2016).

Additional Links:

- https://www.nlm.nih.gov/medlineplus/potassium.html

- http://www.mayoclinic.org/diseases-conditions/muscle-cramp/symptoms-causes/dxc-20186052

- http://www.nationalacademies.org/hmd/Global/News%20Announcements/~/media/442A08B899F44DF9AAD083D86164C75B.ashx

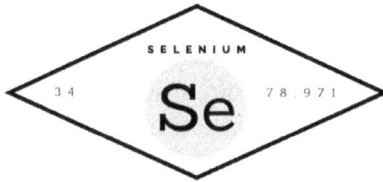

SELENIUM
34   Se   78.971

SELENIUM

Selenium is a natural trace element that can be an essential micronutrient or a toxin, depending on the dose consumed.

Selenium wasn't always known to be an essential nutrient. Prior to the 1950s, veterinary scientists thought it was a toxin because it was related to livestock-related illnesses. This may have been due to an excess of selenium in the soil or in the feed. But in more recent decades, it has become clear to scientists that selenium is needed by animals and humans, and that it may even have anti-cancer effects.

Most of what selenium does or changes in the body is through the action of selenoproteins. These are just what they sound like; proteins that have some selenium in them. Selenium hops into amino acids, creating a special kind of amino acid that attracts oxidation-reduction (free-radical-removing) reactions readily.[1] As you now know, this makes it a great antioxidant, because free radicals cause aging and damage to the body. When you make an enzyme with these selenoproteins, the redox reactions take off!

The supercharged seleno-amino acids make up selenoproteins, which are an important part of antioxidant enzymes like glutathione peroxidase and thioredoxin reductase. They act like building blocks for the enzymes. You can think of them as little Ferrari engines to make all that antioxidant activity go fast.

For example, glutathione peroxidase triggers the conversion of harmful hydrogen peroxide (H_2O_2) to water, preventing the hydrogen peroxide from tearing electrons out of cell membranes and causing cellular damage. Water sounds a lot safer, right?

Thioredoxin reductase is our first line of defense against UV light-caused DNA damage. When UV light hits the skin and starts causing cancer-promoting DNA damage, the thioredoxin is so supercharged by selenium that it neutralizes the DNA damage process. So, people at risk for skin cancer might want to check their selenium levels![2]

DIETARY SOURCES OF SELENIUM

Nutritionists love to tout Brazil nuts for their high selenium content. Just one large nut can have 140 mg of selenium— more than twice the recommended daily amount! Oysters, whole grains and meats also contain selenium.

RECOMMENDED DAILY INTAKE OF SELENIUM

The RDI for selenium in the United States is 55 micrograms per day, with 60 mcg recommended for pregnant women and 70 mcg for lactating women. To show you how much RDIs vary across countries, the Korean standard is 100 mcg per day![7]

SELENIUM DEFICIENCY

While most people in modern nations do not have selenium deficiency, it is a common problem in developing countries. Severe selenium deficiency can cause a weakened heart, male infertility or Kashin-Beck disease, a type of arthritis. Selenium deficiency can increase iodine deficiency as well, making it an important nutrient to test in patients with hypothyroidism.[8]

Pregnant women should be mindful of selenium levels, since deficiency has been associated with preeclampsia, an elevation of high blood pressure that can lead to seizures.[9]

SELENIUM AND CANCER

One of the most intriguing areas of selenium research focuses on the possibility that selenium has cancer-fighting properties. When researchers study groups of people with and without cancer, the groups without cancer certainly seem to have higher selenium levels.

Having healthy selenium levels has been associated with a lower risk of the following cancers: bladder, lung, larynx, prostate, stomach and colon.

Similarly, for stomach cancer, several studies seem to suggest that the risk is lower the higher one's selenium level is.[3] In general, the patients not affected by cancer seemed to have selenium levels between 75 and 150 micrograms per liter, while the cancer patients seemed to have levels of less than 60[4]. This seems to make sense, since we know that selenium is an antioxidant, and antioxidants help to get rid of cellular damage that can lead to cancer.

However, there are two big caveats. One is that these researchers may have been looking at the effect of cancer on selenium levels; the cancer cells may have been "eating up" the selenium for better growth. Another is that, while selenium really might prevent some cancers, giving selenium to someone who already has cancer may backfire. Chemotherapy works because it kills cancer cells, and extra antioxidants can make cancer cells less vulnerable to the damaging effects of chemotherapy.

Two reviews of the medical literature on selenium and cancer concluded that there was no strong evidence to justify people taking selenium specifically to prevent cancer. One was even called "Selenium: Friend or Foe?"[5]

SELENIUM AND THE THYROID

The thyroid gland produces inactive thyroid hormone, which when converted to active thyroid hormone drives the metabolism of the entire body. Thyroid deficiency results in weight gain, mental slowing, and dry skin, among other problems. Selenium helps convert inactive thyroid hormone to active thyroid hormone.

Overall, studies to connect selenium supplements with better thyroid function haven't been conclusive. Some studies show side effects. Other studies, though, suggest that selenium reduces the number of antibodies (immune proteins) that attack the thyroid gland—the culprit in a common low-thyroid disease, Hashimoto's disease. Since the thyroid gland needs to be handled with care in order to avoid serious consequences of too little or not enough supplementation, a well-designed research study will help doctors to know once and for all whether all people with thyroid disease would benefit from extra selenium.[6]

SELENIUM SUPPLEMENTS

Most multivitamins contain selenium. The amount can range from 50 mcg (71 percent of the RDI) to 100 mcg. Some "thyroid supplements" contain much more than the RDI in each pill. If you already get a fair amount of selenium in your diet, it would be wise to assess how much you are getting total before taking a high-selenium supplement. Indeed, the narrow "sweet spot" range for selenium is called the selenium paradox.[7]

EXCESS SELENIUM

Common symptoms of selenium toxicity include a garlicky odor in the breath, fatigue, gastrointestinal symptoms, line marks on the nails, hair loss, and numbness.[10,11]

One study from 2013 looked at toenail clippings (a longer-term assessment of selenium levels than a quick blood snapshot) and found something worrisome; depression symptoms were higher in people who had high levels of selenium accumulation. Specifically, people who had double the average selenium level had a 56 percent higher risk of depression. Another study from New Zealand, which has lower-than-expected rates of selenium intake due to poor content in the soil, found something even more complex; that increased depression rates were found in young people with high and low selenium levels. In fact, the lower the selenium level, the worse the depression.

They found that the optimal range for blood levels, at least in the young adult population studied, was between 82 and 85 µg/L (micrograms per liter) for the lowest risk of depression. This range is interesting because it's also the range of selenium that makes our old friend glutathione peroxidase (remember, the super-antioxidant?) work at maximal efficiency.[12] Because of this, future research on depression will likely look very closely at the role selenium – and oxidative stress – play in depression. Imagine if we could treat depression with selenium monitoring, diet and supplements instead of Prozac and Paxil!

REFERENCES

1. Haas, E. M. & Levin, B. Staying Healthy with Nutrition: The Complete Guide to Diet and Nutritional Medicine. (Celestial Arts, 2006).

2. Patrick, L. Selenium biochemistry and cancer: a review of the literature. Altern Med Rev 9, 239–258 (2004).

3. Gong, H.-Y. et al. Meta-analysis of the association between selenium and gastric cancer risk. Oncotarget 5, (2016).

4. Fritz, H. et al. Selenium and Lung Cancer: A Systematic Review and Meta Analysis. PLoS ONE 6, (2011).

5. Vinceti, M., Crespi, C. M., Malagoli, C., Del Giovane, C. & Krogh, V. Friend or foe? The current epidemiologic evidence on selenium and human cancer risk. J Environ Sci Health C Environ Carcinog Ecotoxicol Rev 31, 305–341 (2013).

6. van Zuuren, E. J., Albusta, A. Y., Fedorowicz, Z., Carter, B. & Pijl, H. Selenium supplementation for Hashimoto's thyroiditis. Cochrane Database Syst Rev CD010223 (2013). doi:10.1002/14651858.CD010223.pub2

7. Lee, K. H. & Jeong, D. Bimodal actions of selenium essential for antioxidant and toxic pro-oxidant activities: the selenium paradox (Review). Mol Med Rep 5, 299–304 (2012).

8. Office of Dietary Supplements - Dietary Supplement Fact Sheet: Selenium. Available at: https://ods.od.nih.gov/factsheets/Selenium-HealthProfessional/. (Accessed: 27th July 2016).

9. Haque, M. M. et al. Low serum selenium concentration is associated with preeclampsia in pregnant women from Bangladesh. Journal of Trace Elements in Medicine and Biology 33, 21–25 (2016).

10. Letavayová, L., Vlcková, V. & Brozmanová, J. Selenium: from cancer prevention to DNA damage. Toxicology 227, 1–14 (2006).

11. Alderman, L. C. & Bergin, J. J. Hydrogen selenide poisoning: an illustrative case with review of the literature. Arch. Environ. Health 41, 354–358 (1986).

12. Conner, T. S., Richardson, A. C. & Miller, J. C. Optimal serum selenium concentrations are associated with lower depressive symptoms and negative mood among young adults. J. Nutr. 145, 59–65 (2015).

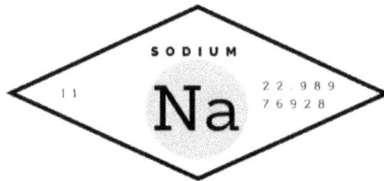

SODIUM

Na

11

22.989
76928

SODIUM

Sodium (chemical name Na) is something we're often told to avoid, but in reality, sodium helps to engineer the actions of every human cell. Every human action—eating, thinking, running, working—depends on adequate sodium. An enzyme in the body pumps sodium and potassium ions across the membranes of every single cell. This pumping of tiny charged atoms creates electrical gradients that power everything that makes us living creatures.

Sodium exists in a delicate balance with both potassium and water. Healthy sodium/potassium and sodium/water balances mean a healthy body, functioning efficiently and effectively. As you will see, imbalances can cause symptoms from mild fatigue to death. However, for most people, there is no need to actively worry about these balances, because our bodies do such a good job of maintaining them. All you need to do is ensure that you don't get too much or too little of good things—sodium, potassium and water. It's not a coincidence that sodium and potassium are the main "electrolytes" that doctors tell you to take while running or when you have a stomach virus.

RECOMMENDED DAILY INTAKE OF SODIUM

In America, the RDI for sodium is 1,500 mg. Pregnant and lactating women require 1,500 mg per day at least. 2,300 mg is the tolerable upper limit for sodium intake.[1]

SODIUM IN FOOD

"Salt" is sodium chloride, the form in which most dietary salt is found, and what is in your salt shaker as well. Low-salt foods are those that contain less than 120 mg of sodium per 100 g of food. Medium-salt foods contain between 120 and 600 mg of sodium per 100 g of food. High-salt foods contain more than 600 mg of sodium per 100 g of food. 100 grams of chicken breast contains about 74 mg of sodium. While that sounds like chicken is a low-sodium food, remember that 100 g is not even as big as a deck of cards—and many restaurant servings are double that![2]

You can find high concentrations of sodium in seafood, meat, processed foods (look at freezer section meals for a real "WOW"), and pickled or brined vegetables like pickles, olives and sauerkraut. Beverages often have a lot of sodium, and even home water softening systems can add too much sodium to drinking water, as it's a replacement for "hardening" agents, like calcium and magnesium.[3]

SODIUM TOXICITY - TWO KINDS

The most basic lab tests include a serum (blood) sodium level. Normal levels are between 135-145 mmol (millimoles per liter). There are two kinds of sodium toxicity: acute and what we call chronic.

Severely restricted water access, not drinking enough water, and some kidney disorders can cause the level of sodium to become acutely too high in the blood, but it's more commonly seen in hospitalized patients, not healthy people just walking around. The "perfect storm" for high sodium would be an elderly patient who does not remember to drink water, who has a kidney disorder, is on diuretics (medicines that make you lose water, usually in order to lower blood pressure) and who is wandering around a desert with no oasis! The symptoms include confusion, weakness and fatigue, and it can lead to seizures. Since a lot of older adults might have the first few symptoms even on a good day, it means that high sodium levels can be easily missed, and can lead to death.[4]

For generally healthy people, though, the sodium/water balancing system is just too good at what it does to allow us to get to that high sodium level. For example, when you eat too much salt, your body automatically retains water to compensate. People tend to notice water retention around their abdomen and in their hands and feet. Plan on going up half a shoe size!

But the body can only rescue you so much, and having to deal with your cheese fries and chips habit can lead to chronic sodium toxicity—the daily burden of your body bailing you out from your own eating, the way the government bailed out bad banks in 2008. Chronically excessive sodium is associated with high blood pressure, and all the negative effects of high blood pressure, and failing kidneys (from the increased work).

SODIUM DEFICIENCY

Low sodium levels in the blood can happen for a number of reasons. These include: drinking far too much water, like a marathon runner guzzling pure water while sweating out all her salt over the course of many hours; not consuming any sodium at all, like people on some fad diets; head injuries; or kidney problems.

Symptoms of low sodium can be similar to that of high sodium, like lethargy, confusion, seizures and death. Nausea and headaches can occur. That's why endurance athletes sometimes need IV fluids after a big race—it's the same treatment people get in the hospital. IV fluids contain sodium with water. Some older people with chronic low sodium have to limit the amount of water they drink in a day or change the medications they take.[5]

When you crave salt, it's often because you're actually dehydrated. Eat a little salty food, and your body will be able to "grab on" to more water instead of letting your kidneys filter it out. Then, drink water!

SODIUM SUPPLEMENTATION

You likely won't find sodium in your multivitamin. That's because it is so ubiquitous in our diets, and because most Americans have the opposite problem—too much. We also get sodium from the many preservatives in our food—sodium phosphate, sodium bicarbonate, and more. Actual sodium tablets are only prescribed in very specific medical situations.

REFERENCES

1. Sodium (Chloride) | Linus Pauling Institute | Oregon State University. Available at: http://lpi.oregonstate.edu/mic/minerals/sodium. (Accessed: 25th October 2016).

2. Sodium - NZ Nutrition Foundation. Available at: http://www.nutritionfoundation.org.nz/nutrition-facts/minerals/sodium. (Accessed: 25th October 2016).

3. Water softeners and sodium - Mayo Clinic. Available at: http://www.mayoclinic.org/healthy-lifestyle/nutrition-and-healthy-eating/expert-answers/water-softeners-sodium/faq-20058469. (Accessed: 25th October 2016).

4. Overgaard-Steensen, C. & Ring, T. Clinical review: practical approach to hyponatraemia and hypernatraemia in critically ill patients. Crit. Care Lond. Engl. 17, 206 (2013).

5. McGreal, K., Budhiraja, P., Jain, N. & Yu, A. S. L. Cu rent Challenges in the Evaluation and Management of Hyponatremia. Kidney Dis. Basel Switz. 2, 56–63 (2016).

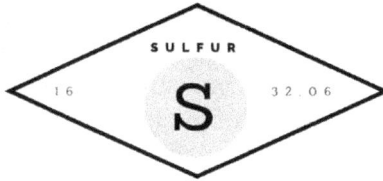

SULFUR

In nature, sulfur is yellow, brittle, odorless and tasteless, and is commonly found near hot springs and volcanic craters. And yes, you read that right – odorless! That rotten egg smell people associate with sulfur is hydrogen sulfide, which is related to sulfur but not the same. In your body, sulfur is the third most abundant mineral, after calcium and phosphorous.

There are many reasons you should know and care about sulfur. Being so abundant in your body, it has many functions. Much of the research about sulfur in the human body is focused on sulfur as an ingredient in organic compounds such as amino acids rather than elemental sulfur.[1,2] Here are just a few examples of sulfur's many uses in the body:

- Homocysteine is a sulfur-containing amino acid, which when found at high levels can be an indicator for certain cardiovascular diseases.
- SAMe is a sulfur-containing substance that can be helpful in people with depression and/or arthritis.
- Glutathione is an excellent antioxidant, which also happens to contain sulfur.
- Chondroitin, glucosamine and methylsulfonylmethane (MSM) are useful supplements for joint pain, and yes, they all contain sulfur.
- Sulfur-containing fibrinogen helps with blood clotting, while sulfur-containing heparin is a blood thinner.
- Sulfonation regulates the activity of steroid hormones (examples: estrogen, testosterone, cortisol and

others), thyroid hormones, bile acids, catecholamines (brain chemicals like dopamine, norepinephrinel, and epinephrine), proper bone structure, cholecystokinin (a hormone that stimulates the digestions of fat and protein), and it also detoxifies certain foreign substances in the body and pharmacological drugs.[5]

- Sulfur is also required for the proper structure and biological activity of enzymes.

DIETARY SOURCES OF SULFUR

Most of your dietary sulfur comes from protein, such as fish, beef and poultry. That's because these foods supply sulfur-containing amino acids like methionine and cysteine. You can also find sulfur in egg yolks, beans, coconut, bananas, pineapple, watermelon, broccoli, garlic, onions, asparagus, leeks, kale, sweet potatoes, peas, chives, avocados, cauliflower, Brussels sprouts, wheat germ and tomatoes.[3]

RECOMMENDED DAILY INTAKE OF SULFUR

Adults need about 6 mg of sulfur-containing amino acids per pound of body weight per day. So you can calculate how much methionine and cysteine you are taking in with your diet and estimate whether you've got enough.[1]

By now, you're sold on why sulfur is a great mineral to have in your body, but let's look more in depth at specific areas where sulfur really shines.

SULFUR AND PREGNANCY

Sulfur-containing methionine is one of those indispensable nutrients required for protein synthesis and the production of SAMe (great for joints and depression). In pregnant women, sulfur levels may be twice as high, in order to supply enough to the developing baby. The kidneys may help by reabsorbing sulfur.

SULFUR AND ANTIMICROBIAL PROPERTIES

A number of sulfur derivatives are successfully used to treat disease-causing germs. Antibiotic classes such as the sulfonamides have been a cornerstone in the treatment of common skin conditions and upper respiratory infections for many decades, going back as far as the 1940s. Sulfur compounds have special capabilities against staphylococcus. Sulfur properties also may help fight some dangerous drug-resistant bacteria, such as MRSA, E.coli and others.[13] DMSO is a sulfur agent that has been FDA-approved for interstitial cystitis (painful bladder syndrome).[14]

SULFUR AND BONE STRUCTURE

People who take sulfur baths (balneotherapy) may see improvements in their strength, have less morning stiffness, have better walking ability, and experience less inflammation, swelling and pain in their joints, particularly in the neck and back, compared to those who don't. Studies of the Dead Sea had similar positive effects on psoriatic arthritis. Sulfur-containing chondroitin and glucosamine[15] are popular supplements,[16] which have beneficial effects on the metabolism of various cells involved in osteoarthritis pain, joint functions, and structure-modifying capacity. Methylsulfonylmethane (MSM) is another common joint pain[17] supplement and may be helpful in reducing pain in people with osteoarthritis. Sulfur-containing polyetheretherketone (PEEK) is used in orthopedic and dental applications because its mechanical properties[18] are similar to those of natural bones.[4]

GLUTATHIONE

This sulfur-containing antioxidant is important for detoxification (getting rid of harmful things in the body like DNA-damaging free radicals). It also regulates cell growth and maintains immune function. Reduced levels of glutathione may be associated with a number of conditions, such as depression, fibromyalgia, arthritis,[20] interstitial cystitis, athletic injuries, congestive heart failure, diabetes, cancer and AIDS.[1]

SULFUR AND MOOD DISORDERS

Sulfur-containing s-adenosylmethionine (SAMe) is a naturally occurring compound found in almost every tissue and fluid in the body. It is involved in many important processes. SAMe plays a role in the immune system, maintains cell membranes, and helps produce and break down brain chemicals, such as serotonin, melatonin, and dopamine. It works with vitamin B12 and folate (vitamin B9). Being deficient in either vitamin B12 or folate may reduce levels of SAMe in your body. SAMe can be beneficial in depression and arthritis.[21]

SULFUR AND SKIN CONDITIONS

Sulfur has antifungal, antibacterial and keratolytic (lesion removing) activity, and is used alone or in combination with agents such as sodium sulfacetamide or salicylic acid. Sulfur is a tried-and-true go-to for many dermatological conditions.[22] It is commonly used to get rid of acne vulgaris, rosacea, eborrheic dermatitis, dandruff, pityriasis versicolor, scabies, warts and human skin mites. Dermatologists sometimes prescribe topical sulfur treatments or sulfur baths.[22-27]

SULFUR AND CANCER

The Allium genus (group) includes garlic, onions, shallots, leeks and chives. Higher intake of these foods has been associated with lower cancer risks. Allium vegetables contain a variety of healthy compounds, including flavonoids, oligosaccharides, arginine and selenium; however, much of Allium's health benefits and the majority of studies on them focus on their sulfur-containing components![29] Studies have shown they may lower your risk of lower gastric and colon cancers, prostate cancer and esophageal cancer. The study that showed the lower risk of esophageal cancer was interesting because all people did was take raw garlic once per week, and their risk was reduced! This is something easy to try, if you can handle the taste! [3,29,30,31]

SULFUR DEFICIENCY

We were unable to find any accurate measurement methods for sulfur deficiency in recent international publications since there are no particular sulfur stores in the body. Sulfur exists in various compounds which may have different concentrations of their own.[7] However, certain groups such as patients with HIV, vegans, athletes and children may be at increased risk for sulfur amino acid deficiencies.[5]

SULFUR SUPPLEMENTATION

Sulfur supplements are not necessary for anyone eating adequate amounts of food, since sulfur is so ubiquitous in nature.

EXCESS SULFUR

Sulfur can cause bad breath (halitosis), but using a mouth rinse or even drinking green tea may help "deodorize" your mouth after a garlic-rich dinner. Generally, coming into contact with sulfur or eating sulfur-rich foods is safe.[33]

REFERENCES

1. Parcell, S. Sulfur in human nutrition and applications in medicine. Altern. Med. Rev. J. Clin. Ther. 7, 22–44 (2002).

2. Baker, D. H. Utilization of isomers and analogs of amino acids and other sulfur-containing compounds. Prog. Food Nutr. Sci. 10, 133–178 (1986).

3. Le Bon, A. M. & Siess, M. H. Organosulfur compounds from Allium and the chemoprevention of cancer. Drug Metabol. Drug Interact. 17, 51–79 (2000).

4. Ouyang, L. et al. Influence of sulfur content on bone formation and antibacterial ability of sulfonated PEEK. Biomaterials 83, 115–126 (2016).

5. Dawson, P. A., Elliott, A. & Bowling, F. G. Sulphate in Pregnancy. Nutrients 7, 1594–1606 (2015).

6. Zlotkin, S. H. & Anderson, G. H. Sulfur balances in intravenously fed infants: effects of cysteine supplementation. Am. J. Clin. Nutr. 36, 862–867 (1982).

7. Golden, M. H. The nature of nutritional deficiency in relation to growth failure and poverty. Acta Paediatr. Scand. Suppl. 374, 95–110 (1991).

8. Kwon, S. W. et al. Prognostic Value of Elevated Homocysteine Levels in Korean Patients with Coronary Artery Disease: A Propensity Score Matched Analysis. Korean Circ. J. 46, 154–160 (2016).

9. Shakhmatova, O. O., Komarov, A. L. & Panchenko, E. P. [Disturbances of homocysteine metabolism as a risk factor of cardiovascular diseases development: effect on prognosis and possibilities of correction with drugs]. Kardiologiia 50, 42–50 (2010).

10. Selhub, J. & Troen, A. M. Sulfur amino acids and atherosclerosis: a role for excess dietary methionine. Ann. N. Y. Acad. Sci. 1363, 18–25 (2016).

11. Tanriverdi, H. et al. Effect of homocysteine-induced oxidative stress on endothelial function in coronary slow-flow. Cardiology 107, 313–320 (2007).

12. Lynch, S. M., Campione, A. L. & Moore, M. K. Plasma thiols inhibit hemin-dependent oxidation of human low-density lipoprotein. Biochim. Biophys. Acta 1485, 11–22 (2000).

13. Weld, J. T. & Gunther, A. THE ANTIBACTERIAL PROPERTIES OF SULFUR. J. Exp. Med. 85, 531–542 (1947).

14. Genç, Y., Özkanca, R. & Bekdemir, Y. Antimicrobial activity of some sulfonamide derivatives on clinical isolates of Staphylococus aureus. Ann. Clin. Microbiol. Antimicrob. 7, 17 (2008).

15. Nasermoaddeli, A. & Kagamimori, S. Balneotherapy in medicine: A review. Environ. Health Prev. Med. 10, 171–179 (2005).

16. Elkayam, O. et al. Immediate and delayed effects of treatment at the Dead Sea in patients with psoriatic arthritis. Rheumatol. Int. 19, 77–82 (2000).

17. Mantovani, V., Maccari, F. & Volpi, N. Chondroitin sulfate and glucosamine as disease modifying anti-osteoarthritis drugs (DMOADs). Curr. Med. Chem. (2016).

18. Kim, L. S., Axelrod, L. J., Howard, P., Buratovich, N. & Waters, R. F. Efficacy of methylsulfonylmethane (MSM) in osteoarthritis pain of the knee: a pilot clinical trial. Osteoarthr. Cartil. OARS Osteoarthr. Res. Soc. 14, 286–294 (2006).

19. Ezaki, J., Hashimoto, M., Hosokawa, Y. & Ishimi, Y. Assessment of safety and efficacy of methylsulfonylmethane on bone and knee joints in osteoarthritis animal model. J. Bone Miner. Metab. 31, 16–25 (2013).

20. Rani, V., Deep, G., Singh, R. K., Palle, K. & Yadav, U. C. S. Oxidative stress and metabolic disorders: Pathogenesis and therapeutic strategies. Life Sci. 148, 183–193 (2016).

21. S-adenosylmethionine. University of Maryland Medical Center Available at: http://umm.edu/health/medical/altmed/supplement/sadenosylmethionine. (Accessed: 1st April 2016).

22. Gupta, A. K. & Nicol, K. The use of sulfur in dermatology. J. Drugs Dermatol. JDD 3, 427–431 (2004).

23. Universtity of Maryland. Sulfur. University of Maryland Medical Center Available at: http://umm.edu/health/medical/altmed/supplement/sulfur. (Accessed: 31st March 2016).

24. Alipour, H. & Goldust, M. The efficacy of oral ivermectin vs. sulfur 10% ointment for the treatment of scabies. Ann. Parasitol. 61, 79–84 (2015).

25. Lin, A. N., Reimer, R. J. & Carter, D. M. Sulfur revisited. J. Am. Acad. Dermatol. 18, 553–558 (1988).

26. Tarimci, N., Sener, S. & Kilinç, T. Topical sodium sulfacetamide/sulfur lotion. J. Clin. Pharm. Ther. 22, 301 (1997).

27. Breneman, D. L. & Ariano, M. C. Successful treatment of acne vulgaris in women with a new topical sodium sulfacetamide/sulfur lotion. Int. J. Dermatol. 32, 365–367 (1993).

28. Li, Y.-M. et al. Dimethyl sulfoxide inhibits zymosan-induced intestinal inflammation and barrier dysfunction. World J. Gastroenterol. 21, 10853–10865 (2015).

29. Milner, J. A. Preclinical perspectives on garlic and cancer. J. Nutr. 136, 827S–831S (2006).

30. Nicastro, H. L., Ross, S. A. & Milner, J. A. Garlic and onions: Their cancer prevention properties. Cancer Prev. Res. Phila. Pa 8, 181–189 (2015).

31. Chen, Y.-K. et al. Food intake and the occurrence of squamous cell carcinoma in different sections of the esophagus in Taiwanese men. Nutr. Burbank Los Angel. Cty. Calif 25, 753–761 (2009).

32. ATSDR - Medical Management Guidelines (MMGs): Sulfur Dioxide. Available at: http://www.atsdr.cdc.gov/mmg/mmg. asp?id=249&tid=46. (Accessed: 1st April 2016).

33. Lodhia, P. et al. Effect of Green Tea on Volatile Sulfur Compounds in Mouth Air. J. Nutr. Sci. Vitaminol. (Tokyo) 54, 89–94 (2008).

34. Cornell University. Sulfur. (1995). Available at: http://pmep.cce. cornell.edu/profiles/extoxnet/pyrethrins-ziram/sulfur-ext.html. (Accessed: 1st April 2016).

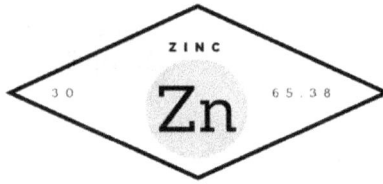

ZINC
30 Zn 65.38

ZINC

You've probably seen zinc lozenges in the cold and flu aisle, but how much do you really know about this essential mineral? As you may have guessed, it is important for a healthy immune system (i.e., it can help you get sick less often or get well quicker!). But that's not all. It's also needed for normal growth and development during pregnancy and childhood, and for men who are zinc deficient, it may even help optimize their testosterone levels.

DIETARY SOURCES OF ZINC

Oysters are the highest source of zinc. But since most people don't eat oysters all the time, the majority of Americans get their zinc from red meat and poultry. You can also get zinc from crabs, shrimp, fish, lobster, oatmeal, whole grains, cheeses, yogurt, beans and nuts.[10]

DAILY RECOMMENDED INTAKE OF ZINC

The recommended daily intake is 11 mg for males, 9 mg for females, 11 mg for pregnant women and 12 mg for lactating women. 2-5 mg is recommended for early childhood.[6]

ZINC DEFICIENCY

Zinc deficiency can be caused by simply not getting enough zinc in your diet,[7] absorption troubles, chronic diseases, and aging. Vegetarians may be at risk due to low meat consumption and because of the phytates in their diets. Phytates are antioxidant compounds found in whole grains, legumes, nuts and seeds, which bind to zinc and make it less absorbable. People with sickle cell disease, chronic alcoholism, lactating women (who lose more zinc), and older adults are more likely to be zinc deficient. Around 1/3 of adults over 60 may have low zinc intake.[13]

Signs and symptoms of zinc deficiency may include loss of appetite, stunted growth in children, sexual immaturity, birth defects, skin problems, dermatitis, diarrhea, poor immune system health, poor healing, altered taste and smell,[21,21] testicular atrophy, hair loss, impotence and mental slowness.[14]

Zinc deficiency can affect both men and women. Having too little or too much zinc may contribute to prostate cancer in men.[15] And, mild zinc deficiency in pregnant women was associated with learning impairments in their children.[16] Zinc deficiency causes an increase in oxidative stress,[17] which basically makes your body more prone to all sorts of health troubles! Increased protein uptake is associated with increased zinc absorption. But note that iron may use the same absorption channels as zinc and, therefore, may interfere with zinc absorption.[13,26]

ZINC DEFICIENCY AND HEART DISEASE

A large analysis revealed that lower zinc levels were associated with more heart attacks.[27]

ZINC DEFICIENCY AND DNA

A study of Ethiopian women with decreased zinc intake revealed that supplementing with 20 mg of zinc for 17 days lead to a decrease in breaks in DNA. These effects are attributed to the role of zinc in reducing oxidative stress. It was noted, though, that zinc plasma levels did not change much, but this is to be expected as the majority of zinc is located in the bones and muscles. Zinc may be a key player in reducing DNA damage.[28,29]

ZINC DEFICIENCY AND NEUROLOGICAL DISEASES

Zinc deficiency and exposure to various metals such as lead, cadmium, arsenic and copper may be linked to psychosis and the development of schizophrenia in early childhood. In a study of 35 patients with uncontrollable epilepsy, researchers found low levels of zinc in 75 percent of the patients, while only 25 percent of healthy controls had zinc deficiency. Another study suggested that zinc supplementation in deficient epileptic people led to an improvement of symptoms. Zinc deficiency also may be a contributor to autism, with low zinc and high copper serum levels.[31-35]

ZINC DEFICIENCY AND BONE HEALTH

The importance of nutrients such as calcium, vitamin D and vitamin K for bone health is well known. However, trace minerals like zinc, copper, fluorine, manganese, magnesium, iron and boron are also important for strong and healthy bones. Deficiencies in these nutrients may lead to slowed bone growth in children, and accelerated bone loss after menopause and in old age.[37]

ZINC DEFICIENCY AND PREGNANCY

Pregnant women may be more likely to become zinc deficient because the fetus diverts some of the mother's zinc. However, zinc is a very important nutrient during this time. Studies have found that miscarriages and preterm deliveries coincided with lower zinc and iron serum blood levels during pregnancy. Zinc is also very important for the baby's neurological development. [40,41-44]

ZINC SUPPLEMENTATION

If you are someone who is likely to be zinc deficient, you can be proactive by getting a blood test to check your zinc levels, and by ensuring zinc is included in your daily multivitamin. If you are zinc deficient, you may benefit from taking a zinc supplement to bring your low zinc levels back to normal. One way to check is through a zinc taste test. You can actually take a mouthful of a liquid zinc supplement to get an idea of how deficient you are. If you don't taste anything, you are deficient. If you do taste it, and it is quite unpleasant, then you are all set.

EXCESS ZINC

You need zinc, but not too much of it. Excess zinc supplementation can lead to copper deficiency and anemia. If large doses of zinc (10–15 times higher than the RDI) are taken by mouth, even for a short period of time, abdominal cramps, nausea, vomiting, diarrhea and headaches may occur.

Ingesting high levels of zinc for several months may cause anemia, damage to the pancreas, and decrease levels of high-density lipoprotein (HDL) cholesterol (the good kind). Zinc toxicity may lead to impaired immune response, hypocupremia, microcytosis, neutropenia, inhibition of copper and iron absorption, respiratory and gastrointestinal toxicity, and inhibition of neurological development.[13,25,26]

REFERENCES

1. Zinc - Element information, properties and uses | Periodic Table. at <http://www.rsc.org/periodic-table/element/30/zinc>

2. Sandstead, H. H. Understanding zinc: recent observations and interpretations. J. Lab. Clin. Med. 124, 322–327 (1994).

3. Terrin, G. & Berni Canani, R. Zinc in Early Life: A Key Element in the Fetus and Preterm Neonate. Nutrients 7, 10427–10446 (2015).

4. Wessells, K. R. & Brown, K. H. Estimating the Global Prevalence of Zinc Deficiency: Results Based on Zinc Availability in National Food Supplies and the Prevalence of Stunting. PLoS ONE 7, (2012).

5. Wastney, M. E., Aamodt, R. L., Rumble, W. F. & Henkin, R. I. Kinetic analysis of zinc metabolism and its regulation in normal humans. Am. J. Physiol. 251, R398–408 (1986).

6. Dietary Reference Intakes for Vitamin A, Vitamin K, Arsenic, Boron, Chromium, Copper, Iodine, Iron, Manganese, Molybdenum, Nickel, Silicon, Vanadium, and Zinc | The National Academies Press. at <http://www.nap.edu/catalog/10026/dietary-reference-intakes-for-vitamin-a-vitamin-k-arsenic-boron-chromium-copper-iodine-iron-manganese-molybdenum-nickel-silicon-vanadium-and-zinc>

7. Briefel, R. R. et al. Zinc Intake of the U.S. Population: Findings from the Third National Health and Nutrition Examination Survey, 1988–1994. J. Nutr. 130, 1367S–1373S (2000).

8. Ervin, R. B. & Kennedy-Stephenson, J. Mineral intakes of elderly adult supplement and non-supplement users in the third national health and nutrition examination survey. J. Nutr. 132, 3422–3427 (2002).

9. Muhamed, P. K. & Vadstrup, S. [Zinc is the most important trace element.]. Ugeskr. Laeger 176, (2014).

10. Office of Dietary Supplements - Zinc. National Institute of Health at <https://ods.od.nih.gov/factsheets/Zinc-HealthProfessional/>

11. World Health Organization. Trace elements in human nutrition and health. (1996). at <apps.who.int/iris/bitstream/10665/37931/2/9241561734_eng.pdf>

12. DEPARTMENT OF HEALTH AND HUMAN SERVICES, Public Health Service & Agency for Toxic Substances and Disease Registry. TOXICOLOGICAL PROFILE FOR ZINC - tp60.pdf. at <http://www.atsdr.cdc.gov/toxprofiles/tp60.pdf>

13. Plum, L. M., Rink, L. & Haase, H. The Essential Toxin: Impact of Zinc on Human Health. Int. J. Environ. Res. Public. Health 7, 1342–1365 (2010).

14. Prasad, A. S. Discovery of human zinc deficiency: its impact on human health and disease. Adv. Nutr. Bethesda Md 4, 176–190 (2013).

15. Singh, B. P. et al. Status and Interrelationship of Zinc, Copper, Iron, Calcium and Selenium in Prostate Cancer. Indian J. Clin. Biochem. IJCB 31, 50–56 (2016).

16. Yu, X. et al. Effects of maternal mild zinc deficiency and different ways of zinc supplementation for offspring on learning and memory. Food Nutr. Res. 60, 29467 (2016).

17. Oteiza, P. I., Clegg, M. S., Zago, M. P. & Keen, C. L. Zinc deficiency induces oxidative stress and AP-1 activation in 3T3 cells. Free Radic. Biol. Med. 28, 1091–1099 (2000).

18. Reed, S. & Neuman, H. Chronic Zinc Deficiency Alters Chick Gut Microbiota Composition and Function. Nutrients 7, 9768–9784 (2015).

19. Kim, S. M. et al. The effect of zinc deficiency on salt taste acuity, preference, and dietary sodium intake in hemodialysis patients. Hemodial. Int. Int. Symp. Home Hemodial. (2016). doi:10.1111/hdi.12388

20. Hsieh, H., Amlal, H. & Genter, M. B. Evaluation of the toxicity of zinc in the rat olfactory neuronal cell line, Odora. Hum. Exp. Toxicol. 34, 308–314 (2015).

21. Jia, H. et al. Enhancement of Odor-Induced Activity in the Canine Brain by Zinc Nanoparticles: A Functional MRI Study in Fully Unrestrained Conscious Dogs. Chem. Senses 41, 53–67 (2016).

22. Bonaventura, P., Lamboux, A., Albarède, F. & Miossec, P. A Feedback Loop between Inflammation and Zn Uptake. PloS One 11, e0147146 (2016).

23. Agency for toxic substances & disease entry. Toxicological Profile: Zinc. Toxicological Profile: Zinc at <http://www.atsdr. cdc.gov/toxprofiles/tp.asp?id=302&tid=54>

24. Fosmire, G. J. Zinc toxicity. Am. J. Clin. Nutr. 51, 225–227 (1990).

25. US National Library of Medicine. TOXNET - Toxicology Data Network. Toxicology Data Network at <http://toxnet.nlm.nih. gov/>

26. Vaz S Silva, S. et al. The impact of water pollution on fish species in southeast region of Goiás, Brazil. J. Toxicol. Environ. Health A 79, 8–16 (2016).

27. Liu, B., Cai, Z.-Q. & Zhou, Y.-M. Deficient zinc levels and myocardial infarction : association between deficient zinc levels and myocardial infarction: a meta-analysis. Biol. Trace Elem. Res. 165, 41–50 (2015).

28. Joray, M. L. et al. Zinc supplementation reduced DNA breaks in Ethiopian women. Nutr. Res. N. Y. N 35, 49–55 (2015).

29. Bai, Y. et al. Essential Metals Zinc, Selenium, and Strontium Protect against Chromosome Damage Caused by Polycyclic Aromatic Hydrocarbons Exposure. Environ. Sci. Technol. 50, 951–960 (2016).

30. Hamza, R. T., Hamed, A. I. & Sallam, M. T. Effect of zinc supplementation on growth hormone-insulin growth factor axis in short Egyptian children with zinc deficiency. Ital. J. Pediatr. 38, 21 (2012).

31. Modabbernia, A., Arora, M. & Reichenberg, A. Environmental exposure to metals, neurodevelopment, and psychosis. Curr. Opin. Pediatr. (2016). doi:10.1097/MOP.0000000000000332

32. Kheradmand, Z. et al. Comparison of Serum Zinc and Copper levels in Children and adolescents with Intractable and Controlled Epilepsy. Iran. J. Child Neurol. 8, 49–54 (2014).

33. Mortazavi, M. et al. Efficacy of Zinc Sulfate as an Add-on Therapy to Risperidone Versus Risperidone Alone in Patients With Schizophrenia: A Double-Blind Randomized Placebo-Controlled Trial. Iran. J. Psychiatry Behav. Sci. 9, e853 (2015).

34. Liu, T. et al. Comparative Study on Serum Levels of 10 Trace Elements in Schizophrenia. PloS One 10, e0133622 (2015).

35. Grabrucker, S., Jannetti, L. & Eckert, M. Zinc deficiency dysregulates the synaptic ProSAP/Shank scaffold and might contribute to autism spectrum disorders. Brain J. Neurol. 137, 137–152 (2014).

36. SAYEHMIRI, F. et al. Zn/Cu Levels in the Field of Autism Disorders: A Systematic Review and Meta-analysis. Iran. J. Child Neurol. 9, 1–9 (2015).

37. Zofková, I., Nemcikova, P. & Matucha, P. Trace elements and bone health. Clin. Chem. Lab. Med. 51, 1555–1561 (2013).

38. Foster, M., Chu, A., Petocz, P. & Samman, S. Effect of vegetarian diets on zinc status: a systematic review and meta-analysis of studies in humans. J. Sci. Food Agric. 93, 2362–2371 (2013).

39. Foster, M. & Samman, S. Vegetarian diets across the lifecycle: impact on zinc intake and status. Adv. Food Nutr. Res. 74, 93–131 (2015).

40. Shen, P.-J., Gong, B., Xu, F.-Y. & Luo, Y. Four trace elements in pregnant women and their relationships with adverse pregnancy outcomes. Eur. Rev. Med. Pharmacol. Sci. 19, 4690–4697 (2015).

41. Liu, K., Mao, X., Shi, J., Lu, Y. & Liu, C. Evaluation of lead and essential elements in whole blood during pregnancy: a cross-sectional study. Ir. J. Med. Sci. (2015). doi:10.1007/s11845-015-1339-9

42. Bailey, R. L., West, K. P. & Black, R. E. The epidemiology of global micronutrient deficiencies. Ann. Nutr. Metab. 66 Suppl 2, 22–33 (2015).

43. Darnton-Hill, I. & Mkparu, U. C. Micronutrients in Pregnancy in Low- and Middle-Income Countries. Nutrients 7, 1744–1768 (2015).

44. Imdad, A., Bhutta, Z. A. & Nestle. Intervention strategies to address multiple micronutrient deficiencies in pregnancy and early childhood. Nestlé Nutr. Inst. Workshop Ser. 70, 61–73 (2012).

45. Haase, H. & Rink, L. Zinc signals and immune function. BioFactors Oxf. Engl. 40, 27–40 (2014).

46. Caulfield, Laura & World Health Organization. in (World Health Organization). at <http://www.who.int/publications/cra/chapters/volume1/0257-0280.pdf>

47. Bonaventura, P., Benedetti, G., Albarède, F. & Miossec, P. Zinc and its role in immunity and inflammation. Autoimmun. Rev. 14, 277–285 (2015).

48. Mocchegiani, E. et al. Zinc: dietary intake and impact of supplementation on immune function in elderly. Age Dordr. Neth. 35, 839–860 (2013).

PART III

YOUR LIFESTYLE
AND MINERALS

LIFESTYLE CHOICES THAT CONTRIBUTE TO MINERAL DEFICIENCY

SODAS

Phosphoric acid is used to enhance the flavor of many carbonated drinks. It provides that tanginess that we enjoy. Although phosphorus is an integral part of bones, high phosphorous intake, such as from the acidic forms found in sodas, can cause essential healthy bone minerals such as calcium and magnesium to get pushed away while phosphates take their place leading to brittle bones (osteoporosis).[1,2]

ALCOHOL

Chronic excessive alcohol users frequently have multiple nutritional and mineral deficits.[3,4] Alcohol has strong diuretic effects which may contribute to loss of minerals in the urine. There are other mechanisms by which alcohol depletes minerals and affects bone formation. These are complex and technical issues, which are beyond the scope of this book and will not be addressed.[5]

COFFEE

In some older studies, increased coffee intake was mentioned as a minor contributor to osteoporosis;[6] recent studies did not find any differences.[7] It is also noteworthy that different types of coffee contain different amounts of minerals.[6] Overall, regular use of one cup of coffee per day does not seem to have any adverse effects on minerals and bone health, while high use may.

WATER WITH LOW MINERAL CONTENT

The minerals in drinking water from a municipal source or from bottled water differ.[9,10] Clinical studies suggest that drinking water that is rich in bicarbonate and potassium lowered calcium excretion in the urine and bone resorption.[11] That means bone is being better preserved. Mineral waters rich in potassium, magnesium, medium calcium and low sodium content are useful for overall health not just for bone and cardiovascular benefits. Fluids lacking in minerals may be counterproductive to health.[11]

STRESS

Stress increases cortisol levels and also interferes with other mineral-reabsorbing hormones. This may cause increased urinary frequency, decreased mineral absorption and loss of essential minerals.[12]

LACK OF MINERAL-RICH FOODS

Many individuals may be lacking in minerals because they do not eat foods that are rich in minerals. It is generally difficult to see the results of such mineral deficits because the clinical signs may be vague and nonspecific. For example, some of the short term clinical signs of mineral deficiencies may be rather nonspecific, such as fatigue, appetite changes, constipation, headaches, sleep disturbances, muscle tightness and cramps, changes in menstruation and premenstrual syndromes, hair loss, skin conditions, memory and concentration issues, to name few.

Long-term clinical signs of mineral deficiencies may include more profound disturbances as noted, and can contribute to a large variety of chronic disabling conditions such as heart disease, brittle bones, disorders of the immune system, developmental disorders in children and premature aging. In the U.S., the most common mineral deficits include iron, magnesium, potassium and zinc.

OTHER CAUSES OF MINERAL DEFICIENCY

Malabsorption in the gastrointestinal tract

This can occur due to a number of inflammatory illnesses and conditions as well as surgery.

Most common causes of malabsorption are:

- Colitis or Crohn's disease
- Gluten allergy and intolerance
- Gastrointestinal infections by bacteria, viruses and parasites
- Surgical removal of bowel loops due to acute emergencies as well as bypass surgeries for weight loss

REFERENCES

1. Takeda, E., Yamamoto, H., Yamanaka-Okumura, H. & Taketani, Y. Increasing dietary phosphorus intake from food additives: potential for negative impact on bone health. Adv. Nutr. Bethesda Md 5, 92–97 (2014).

2. Calvo, M. S. & Tucker, K. L. Is phosphorus intake that exceeds dietary requirements a risk factor in bone health? Ann. N. Y. Acad. Sci. 1301, 29–35 (2013).

3. González-Reimers, E. et al. Prognosis of osteopenia in chronic alcoholics. Alcohol Fayettev. N 45, 227–238 (2011).

4. Mikosch, P. Alcohol and bone. Wien. Med. Wochenschr. 1946 164, 15–24 (2014).

5. Maurel, D. B., Boisseau, N., Benhamou, C. L. & Jaffre, C. Alcohol and bone: review of dose effects and mechanisms. Osteoporos. Int. J. Establ. Result Coop. Eur. Found. Osteoporos. Natl. Osteoporos. Found. USA 23, 1–16 (2012).

6. Johansson, C., Mellström, D., Lerner, U. & Osterberg, T. Coffee drinking: a minor risk factor for bone loss and fractures. Age Ageing 21, 20–26 (1992).

7. Kim, S. Y. Coffee Consumption and Risk of Osteoporosis. Korean J. Fam. Med. 35, 1 (2014).

8. Hallström, H. et al. Long-term coffee consumption in relation to fracture risk and bone mineral density in women. Am. J. Epidemiol. 178, 898–909 (2013).

9. Petraccia, L., Liberati, G., Masciullo, S. G., Grassi, M. & Fraioli, A. Water, mineral waters and health. Clin. Nutr. Edinb. Scotl. 25, 377–385 (2006).

10. Garzon, P. & Eisenberg, M. J. Variation in the mineral content of commercially available bottled waters: implications for health and disease. Am. J. Med. 105, 125–130 (1998).

11. Burckhardt, P. [Mineral waters and bone health]. Rev. Médicale Suisse Romande 124, 101–103 (2004).

12. Herman, J. P. et al. Regulation of the Hypothalamic-Pituitary-Adrenocortical Stress Response. Compr. Physiol. 6, 603–621 (2016).

13. NIH. Magnesium Fact Sheet. National Institute of Health Available at: https://ods.od.nih.gov/factsheets/Magnesium-HealthProfessional/.

14. National Institue of Health. Potassium in diet: MedlinePlus Medical Encyclopedia. Available at: https://www.nlm.nih.gov/medlineplus/ency/article/002413.htm. (Accessed: 24th February 2016).

15. Dietary Sources of Iron - McKinley Health Center - University of Illinois. Available at: http://www.mckinley.illinois.edu/handouts/dietary_sources_iron.html. (Accessed: 22nd April 2016).

WHY ROUTINE DOCTOR TESTING MAY NOT BE ENOUGH

It should be simple enough to have your doctor do a blood test and get an answer as to whether your mineral levels are too low or too high. The real problem is that many doctors do not routinely test for certain mineral deficiencies. Usually your doctor will order a "chem panel" (Comprehensive Metabolic Panel). This panel includes common minerals such as potassium (K), sodium (Na), calcium (Ca) and chlorine (Cl). The blood is drawn, spun in a centrifuge to separate blood cells from the serum and ONLY the serum minerals get measured. That's the base test. You might get some tests for iron levels, rarely a magnesium level and that's pretty much it. Important other minerals like zinc or trace minerals such as manganese, selenium, chromium or sulfur-containing amino acids are rarely ever tested. So, you may not find out about important mineral deficiencies unless you take the time to educate yourself and request those tests or see a practitioner familiar with mineral testing.

SO HOW CAN MINERALS BE TESTED?

Minerals can be tested in blood plasma, urine, hair, tissue biopsies and proteins that specifically carry certain minerals.

MINERALS TESTED IN BLOOD SERUM

Blood serum levels for sodium, potassium, zinc and magnesium are easy to check. However, there may be circumstances where you may need different tests other than simply checking minerals swimming in your blood vessels. For example, you may need to test potassium and magnesium inside the blood cells. Why? There are many instances where blood tests will register as normal when the mineral test is done in the serum, but register as abnormal when tested inside the blood cells. In other words, you can have an intracellular mineral deficit and a normal extracellular mineral concentration. So basically, the regular blood test at your doctor's office might show a normal result for potassium or magnesium, while the cells themselves do not have enough of them inside the cell. Potassium and magnesium measurement from red blood cells can more accurately evaluate whether a deficit exists.

If you want better answers for your potassium or magnesium status, ask for potassium RBC or magnesium RBC.

MINERAL TESTED INDIRECTLY BY CARRIER OR STORAGE PROTEINS

Some minerals are tested indirectly by checking proteins to which they are usually bound. Measuring your iron (Fe) level may not detect an iron deficiency since iron is more often bound to a particular protein called ferritin which helps to store iron in the body and is also in circulation in the blood.[1] There is another protein that transports iron called transferrin. We can measure how much iron transferrin carries and if the load is low, you are likely to be low in iron.[1] Zinc levels can also be tested by measuring its carrier protein, ceruloplasmin.

MINERALS ARE NOT EQUALLY DISTRIBUTED IN THE HUMAN BODY

Calcium and phosphorus are mostly stored in bones; therefore, calcium plasma levels do not reflect the total body reserve of these minerals. Estimating calcium and phosphorous in bones is better done by bone scans.

Similarly, 90 percent of total body zinc is stored in muscles and bones. Therefore, other analysis samples, such as hair, can be evaluated in addition to blood levels.

TESTING TRACE MINERALS

Low amounts of iodine[3], selenium[4], manganese[5], molybdenum and chromium are present in the human body, but they are critical for various biochemical reactions, and enzymatic and antioxidant functions. Iodine levels in the blood are not commonly tested, because of very low levels.

A more commonly used test is to analyze iodine urine concentrations. Selenium, manganese, molybdenum and chromium testing can be done by blood draws. There are also other ways of testing minerals in regards to their functional impact. For example, selenium is a crucial component for an important enzyme (glutathione peroxidase). If this enzyme is low, it commonly correlates with a functional selenium deficit.[6]

TESTING FOR CHEMICAL COMPOUNDS RATHER THAN ISOLATED MINERAL TESTING

Sulfur is distributed in varying concentrations throughout the body.[7] In this scenario, it is most useful to test for important biochemical compounds such as sulfa-containing amino acids. Amino acids are building blocks for many proteins and enzymes. Glutathione is an important sulfa compound that helps the body's immune system, is a powerful antioxidant, and fights toxins and damages to the body.

OTHER TEST ISSUES

Inflammation

Blood concentration of minerals may change depending on varying degrees of inflammation in the body and cells. Certain minerals absorb and circulate in the blood differently during inflammatory states. A key inflammation marker, C-reactive protein, may be helpful to interpret your mineral results.[8,9]

Lab Errors

Sometimes, normal individuals may get an abnormally high potassium reading. This may be due to either an extended traumatic blood draw or prolonged storage issues.[10] Blood cells will generally break down and release intracellular potassium in the serum. Repeating the test can determine whether the error is related to a defective machine or technique.

SUMMARY

Symptoms for mineral deficiency can be vague and nonspecific, and it may not be easy for you to know that you have a mineral deficit. Skilled medical practitioners may suspect certain deficiencies, but they have to rely on testing to confirm. Furthermore, mineral deficiencies are more likely to affect people over 40 years. It generally takes a long time for the effects of mineral deficits to manifest themselves in healthy people. It is therefore important to be proactive and routinely test for nutrients. Understanding and testing for deficiencies during childhood is also important since these mineral deficiencies can lead to a number of developmental disorders or impairments. In addition, choose a knowledgeable expert to interpret your mineral test results.

REFERENCES

1. How Is Iron-Deficiency Anemia Diagnosed? - NHLBI, NIH. Available at: http://www.nhlbi.nih.gov/health/health-topics/topics/ida/diagnosis. (Accessed: 27th April 2016).

2. Wastney, M. E., Aamodt, R. L., Rumble, W. F. & Henkin, R. I. Kinetic analysis of zinc metabolism and its regulation in normal humans. Am. J. Physiol. 251, R398-408 (1986).

3. ZRT laboratory. Iodine Deficiency. Available at: http://www.zrtlab.com/health-concerns/iodine-deficiency. (Accessed: 27th April 2016).

4. NIH. Selenium Fact sheet. Available at: https://ods.od.nih.gov/factsheets/Selenium-HealthProfessional/. (Accessed: 20th January 2016).

5. University of Maryland. Manganese. University of Maryland Medical Center Available at: http://umm.edu/health/medical/altmed/supplement/manganese. (Accessed: 16th March 2016).

6. SES - Clinical: Selenium, Serum. Available at: http://www.mayomedicallaboratories.com/test-catalog/Clinical+and+Interpretive/9765. (Accessed: 16th September 2016).

7. Universtity of Maryland. Sulfur. University of Maryland Medical Center Available at: http://umm.edu/health/medical/altmed/supplement/sulfur. (Accessed: 31st March 2016).

8. Salota, R., Omar, S., Sherwood, R. A., Raja, K. & Vincent, R. P. Clinical relevance of trace element measurement in patients on initiation of parenteral nutrition. Ann. Clin. Biochem. (2016). doi:10.1177/0004563216633489

9. Shenkin, A. Trace elements and inflammatory response: implications for nutritional support. Nutr. Burbank Los Angel. Cty. Calif 11, 100–105 (1995).

10. Khodorkovsky, B., Cambria, B., Lesser, M. & Hahn, B. Do hemolyzed potassium specimens need to be repeated? J. Emerg. Med. 47, 313–317 (2014).

WHERE TO HAVE YOUR MINERAL LEVELS CHECKED

Throughout this guide to being proactive with minerals to get and stay healthy, we have recommended getting your mineral levels tested to identify any potential deficiencies or imbalances. To get this testing, you should first check with your health care provider to see if he or she offers this service and, if so, how comprehensive the test will be. If your health care provider doesn't offer full-spectrum mineral testing, you can easily get this test by contacting:

PROACTIVE HEALTH LABS

If you are in Southern California, we would be delighted to provide mineral testing and counsel you on the results and steps you can take to get and stay your healthiest. Learn more about us by visiting **phlabs.org**, or call **855-PHLABS1**.

If you would prefer to go to a local lab near you, here are some of the best options for you:

SPECTRACELL MICRONUTRIENT TEST

Find a draw site near you at https://www.spectracell.com/clinicians/find-a-draw-site/. Or call Spectracell at 800-227-5227.

GENOVA DIAGNOSTICS NUTREVAL TEST

Email Genova to find partnering doctors near you at https://www.gdx.net/patients/find-a-doctor. Or call Genova at 800-522-4762.

QUEST DIAGNOSTICS

Quest Diagnostics offers tests for specific minerals, but they must be ordered through your doctor's office. If you are unsure of which test you want to request, you can call 866-MYQUEST and select Option 2 to speak with Quest's customer service.

Your doctor may draw your blood in the office or send you to a Quest lab. To find out if they have a lab near you, go to QuestDiagnostics.com, look under the For Patients tab, and select Find a Location. Or go directly to this link: https://secure.questdiagnostics.com/hcp/psc/jsp/SearchLocation.do?newSearch=FindLocation.

Enjoy your healthy life!

PART IV

THE pH LABS
EDITORIAL BOARD

"MINERALS: The Forgotten Nutrient" is based on pH's approach for getting and staying your healthiest. It was researched and written in close cooperation with recognized, leading experts from the medical and legal fields at pH. Contributing editors for this book were all members of the pH Labs health care team.

JOY STEPHENSON-LAWS, JD

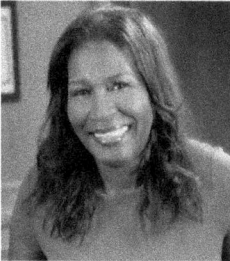

Joy Stephenson-Laws is the founder of Proactive Health Labs (pH), a revolutionary health care company that provides consumers with the information and tools they need to achieve optimal health.

Ms. Stephenson-Law's commitment to enhancing consumer health and positively impacting the health care industry is not new and goes beyond her work as a health care attorney. In fact, both her professional and personal lives have been dedicated to improving health care in the United States, from consumer education to being an advocate for health care providers, and from founding a health care-related philanthropy to encouraging others to get involved in their communities.

Her passion for motivating people to proactively protect their health comes from her personal experience of losing loved ones, colleagues and friends to diseases which, had they been diagnosed early enough and treated more effectively, could either have been controlled or cured.

In addition to her day-to-day leadership role with pH, Ms. Stephenson-Laws is also the founding and managing partner of Stephenson, Acquisto & Colman (SAC), the health care industry's premier litigation law firm established in 1989. She also is co-founder and president of MoJo Marketing & Media, a company dedicated to developing ways for individuals and companies to give back to their communities through sports and entertainment. Ms. Stephenson-Laws also co-founded the Bili-Project, a nonprofit organization that is driving funding and research for identifying markers for biliary cancer so that this leading cause of cancer deaths in the United States can be more effectively diagnosed and treated.

Ms. Stephenson-Laws received her B.A. from Loma Linda University in 1980 and Juris Doctor from Loyola University in 1983, and was admitted to the California Bar in 1984. Professional organizations include the American Bar Association, Consumer Attorneys of Los Angeles, California State Bar Association, U.S. District Court-Central/Eastern, and Ninth Circuit Court of Appeals.

MONYA DE, MD, MPH

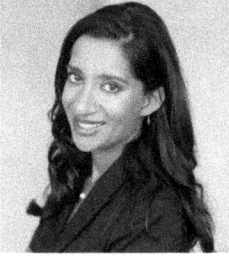

Dr. De is a specialist in internal medicine and previously was a medical reporter for ABC News. Dr. De was graduated with her MPH degree from the University of California, Berkeley School of Public Health and her MD degree from the University of California, Irvine. She received her undergraduate degree with honors in human biology from Stanford University. Dr. De is a proponent of integrative medicine and works with patients to prioritize the most natural way to heal and to prevent disease even before symptoms develop. Dr. De's work has borne out her conviction that many symptoms do not need a prescription but can be readily addressed by ensuring that our bodies have the ideal amount and balance of nutrients, including minerals, that they need to be their healthiest. In addition to her medical and health-related work, Dr. De is an avid scuba diver and practitioner of yoga.

FRANZ GLIEDERER, MD, MPH

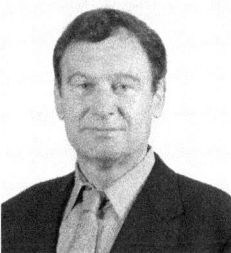

Dr. Gliederer is a specialist in preventive medicine with a Medical Doctorate from the University of Vienna, Austria and a master's degree from the University of California Public Health School. Dr. G has a diverse medical background including three residencies in occupational and preventive medicine at the University of Southern California Los Angeles, internal medicine at St. Joseph Medical Center in Chicago, and family medicine in Vienna, Austria as well as working two decades in urgent care/ER, occupational medicine, and integrative medicine. He was also a published research fellow at the Pulmonary Division of UCLA. Dr.G is committed to advancing and helping people to take a more proactive, preventive approach to getting and staying their healthiest. Privately, he has been an accomplished competitive athlete in track, shotokan karate and golf, as well as a published photographer and a contributor to travel lifestyle magazines.

PAULINE J. JOSE, MD

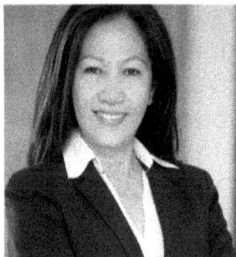

Dr. Jose is a member of the Cedars-Sinai Medical Center staff in Los Angeles, California. She is also a clinical instructor at UCLA, Department of Family Medicine. She received her MD degree from the University of the East, Ramon Magsaysay Memorial Medical Center in Manila, the Philippines and her BA degree from the University of the Philippines in Quezon City, the Philippines. Dr. Jose completed her residency in family medicine at the Brooklyn Hospital Center in Brooklyn, New York. Dr. Jose is a firm believer of practicing the advice she gives her patients at pH Labs by identifying her own vitamin and mineral deficiencies and taking supplements to ensure she has the right balance to be her healthiest. Dr. Jose loves sports, dancing and traveling.

DISCLOSURE

The contents of this book are for informational purposes only and do not constitute medical advice. It is not intended to be a substitute for professional medical advice, diagnosis, or treatment. Always seek the advice of a physician or other qualified health provider with any questions you may have regarding a medical condition. Never disregard professional medical advice or delay in seeking it because of something you have read in this book.

www.ingramcontent.com/pod-product-compliance
Lightning Source LLC
Chambersburg PA
CBHW052130270326
41930CB00012B/2824